Non-Alcoholic Fatty Liver Disease

Liver Cleanse Diet & Recipes

because a happier liver makes a happier life!

Copyright

All rights reserved. No part of this book may be reproduced or transmitted in any form or by any means, electronic or mechanical, including photocopying, recording or by any information storage and retrieval system, without permission in writing from the author.

This book is not intended as a substitute for the medical advice of physicians. The reader should regularly consult a physician in matters relating to his/her health and particularly with respect to any symptoms or medication that may require diagnosis or medical attention.

If you have a medical condition that requires you to eat a particular product, you should consult your doctor before making any changes.

Rossano, Diana Jo, Ph.D.

Non-Alcoholic Fatty Liver Disease Liver Cleanse Diet & Recipes because a happier liver makes a happier life!

All rights reserved © Copyright 2010, 2013, 2015 by Diana Jo Rossano, Ph.D.

Photographic Credit: Pil McNiff

Table of Contents

Copyright iii
Table of Contents v
Acknowledgements vii
Mary Beat Fatty Liver Disease 9
Cleansing Your Liver 11
Liver Cleanse – One-Week Plan 19
Liver Cleanse – Six-Week Plan 25
The "Lazy, Sneaky Cook" Tells All! 31
Liver Cleanse Diet Foundation 43
Healthy Hearsay 57
Food as Medicine 67
My Discovery 75
Bad Fats & Oils, Enemy #1 81
Sugar, Liver Enemy #2 97
Enriched Foods, Liver, Enemy #3 103
Chemicals, Enemy #4 109
Animal Products, Enemy #5 133
Emotional Problems 151
Case Study - Bipolar Disorder 155
Case Study – Hypoglycemia 163
Case Study – Anxiety Attack 167
Case Study - Drug/Alcohol Abuse 171
Case Study - Migraines 177
Case Study – Painful Leg Cramps and Sore Feet 181
Magician in the Kitchen 185

Eating Out Without Being Killed 189

Recipe Section 199

Dr. B's Recipe 345

Home Canning Information 346

Snack Choices 355

Drink Choices 357

Substitutes for Recipes 367

Substitutes More 373

Herbal Liver Medicine – Milk Thistle 377

Planning a Simple Party 379

Addendum: 21 Ways to Love Your Liver 381

Addendum: Adapting your Recipes 405

Addendum: Fruit - the easiest and best breakfast 407

Addendum: Planning a Family Outing 409

Addendum: Relapse Insurance 411

Addendum: Getting a Good Night's Rest 417

About the Author 419

Bibliography 423

Index for Recipes 427

Acknowledgements

The Good Book says,

"The Rock of my strength and my refuge is God."

Psalm 62:7

Thanks to God for healing me from migraine headaches, ulcerative colitis, hypoglycemia, low thyroid, fibromyalgia and TMJ. My doctors (yes - plural - - lots of doctors) suggested that I take prescription pain medication everyday to "control" my pain.

I did NOT want a normal life of taking prescription pain medication every day. What did I do? In 1995, I started my research to find out the reason for my body was having so much pain.

That research brought me back to school. Today, my illnesses are in complete remission! The pages that follow are my research. This research may give you the education you need to understand why the recipes contain the ingredients I have chosen.

Mary Beat Fatty Liver Disease

Mary had survived breast cancer for the second time when I met her. She was approximately 55 years of age and was worried about her fatty liver disease. Every time she went to see her oncologist for a check up, he would sadly wag his head when he reported her blood work findings, "I'm sorry, Mary, but your blood work still shows you have a fatty liver."

I suggested that Mary purchase my book "<u>Feel Better in 48 Hours Plan</u>." This book is no longer in print, but I have completely revised it to become this book.

Mary followed the book as if her life depended on it. At her very next check up with her oncologist - - about three months later - - her fatty liver disease was gone. Yes, I said gone - in complete remission. All of her blood work came back completely normal. Mary said, "YAY!"

Mary has had her energy increase, she lost about three pounds. (Her weight was normal for her age and height.)

Congratulations! You have found the right tool in your hands to help your body to improve the health of your liver. YES, you can improve liver diseases, but it will take some planning by you. This is a complete lifestyle change to many of my students. But, be encouraged you can do this if you move slowly. Slow and steady will win the race to achieve health for your liver. When your liver enzyme test comes back normal, please go to my website and share the good news or write me a review of this book on Amazon. Thank you.

Cleansing Your Liver

Let's talk about cleansing your liver for the first step to jump start your journey to better health. Mary did NOT go through this cleansing step. She was working a full-time job and her schedule would not allow her to take time off from work.
You have options:

1) Skip this first detoxification step and go right to the six-week plan and once a week do one of the liver treatments. The liver treatments are in the addendum of this book. Please check the index at the back of the book.

OR

2) Use the one week cleanse to kick start your healing and then start eating from the recipe plan along with one liver treatment each week. Please refrain from eating out until you get a good report.

OR

3) The Six-Week Plan to allow you to ease yourself into eating an entirely different way than most people in America eat. On the other hand, if you went to the doctor and had a liver enzyme test or ultra sound that diagnosed you with Non Fatty Liver disease, then the cleansing may prove to be beneficial to you.

If you get a headache, feel more tired than usual, **then slow down** the cleansing suggestions. Don't be upset because your liver is able to heal itself if you give it the correct tools for repair. The headache or feeling tired, is feedback from your body that you want to clean house faster than your liver is able to clean.

It took you a long time of eating unhealthy to be where you are today, so give your liver some time to reverse all those years of mistaken eating habits. Fatty liver syndrome simply means that your liver isn't burning fat, but storing fat.

Your liver is NOT designed to store fat. This problem has happened to you because you are eating the bad fats and additives in your diet for a extended time.

Most people think that having liver disease means they need to start eating low fat or no fat foods. This is <u>WRONG</u>! In fact, the low fat and no fat foods contain bad fats. Bad fats are one of the main contributing causes to why your liver is fatty. You may think you are eating a remedy, but you are eating one of the contributing causes of your liver health problem.

It would be like a cocaine addict trying to kick his habit by doing more cocaine. Of course, Food Manufacturers don't tell you that low fat and no fat foods aren't healthy—- why would they tell you and ruin their profitable business? Never.

Instead, Food Manufacturers write "buzz words" that you want to see on the front of their labels. You quickly purchase their food product with the right buzz words. I call this "Healthy Hearsay." More on this later. This is a money thing and nothing else. They do NOT want to hurt you. They just want to dip their hand in your pocket for your donation – that's it.

Your liver is in charge of your immune system. Your liver helps you to LIVE. Just add one letter "R" and you have liveR. Since your liver is the General of your immune system, it would be like commanding the troops (white blood cells, killer cells, etc.) how to fight disease without the General (liver.)

If the General is defeated, the troops fail to fight disease and being sick wins the battle. Eventually, if your immune system doesn't fight, you will have an increased chance of developing a dangerous disease like cancer. I have a book called, "What Causes Cancer, Processed Foods to Avoid" for friends and family who want help. this book will do the same thing. What? Avoid cancer. Yes, eating the recipes in this book may help you to avoid cancer.

Deadly Deeds that Deaden your liver:

- Eating refined white sugar is toxic to your liver.
- Fumes from using cleaners, painting, exhaust and other environmental contact contribute to inflammation of the liver.
- Cholesterol-lowering drugs are detrimental to the liver.
- ALL prescription medication are toxic to your liver.
- ALL over-the-counter (OTC) drugs are toxic to your liver.
- Drinking one alcoholic drink per day is a diuretic and robs your body of water. Less water means your liver is handicapped to clean itself.

- Drinking water from plastic containers because plastic outgases BPA or bisphenol A which is a type of woman's hormone called, "estrogen."

- Not drinking good, clean water. Tap water is deadly because of the fluoride added to it. No, 90 percent of water filters won't remove fluoride. I highly suggest a distillery for drinking and cooking water. More on this later.

- Eating processed foods that have food coloring & other additives. If your food is in a jar, can, box, bag or anything that has a label – it is a processed food. You must become your own food processor.

- HRT (hormone replacement therapy)

- Birth control pills

- Drinking tap water that has chlorine, fluoride and other contaminants in it. See my website for water filter suggestions: http://www.migrainephd.com/water/

- Cooking food in a microwave oven for longer than three minutes. Please know, I do NOT own a microwave.

- Eating vitamins—if it is a pill, it's not natural to a human body - no matter what the label says. Please eat food made from the good of the land and not anything made by man.

- Drinking Health Shakes—check the long ingredient list for words that are chemicals. Please don't eat chemicals. Just because the label says, "Health" shake, doesn't mean it is healthy for you. The shake makes the food manufacturer have a healthier bank account is a true statement.

- Some health care providers suggest using chemicals to cleanse your liver. This only makes sense if you sell the chemicals for a profit.

Fatty liver diseases are on the rise. Most Americans think that this disease is limited to people who drink alcohol. Well, think again. According to Dr. Robert H. Lustig, M.D., the definition of a poison would be any chemical that can only be metabolized by the liver.

Eating fructose corn syrup in your food is NOT natural to the body and the body can only metabolize fructose when it cycled in the blood into the liver for filtering. That makes high fructose corn syrup a poison to your liver.

These are some of the contributing causes to liver disease. Can the body metabolize hydrolyzed vegetable protein? Partially hydrogenated oil? MSG? Monosodium glutamate or other chemicals that are in our food?

Yes, a person may be able to metabolize these chemicals if they have a strong liver. While a person is young and the liver is clean and healthy, the liver has a good chance that it can clean some of these chemicals out of the blood. As the person ages, well. . . .that becomes a different story.

In my own life, I could eat a mayonnaise sandwich (deadly) and the next day, I was fine. As I aged and my liver was busy trying to remove all the NON food chemicals I was eating, that's when I developed headaches. I always thought my headaches were caused by something blooming in the air – you know – an allergy.

In reality, my headaches were caused by eating the wrong foods from the above list. If you think of your liver as a filter – because that is one of its 400 jobs, then don't clog the filter with additives and preservatives. Your liver cleans your blood.

Exercise is beneficial for everyone's health because the extra activity forces the blood through the liver more often than a couch potato. The blood's faster traveling through the liver caused by exercising gives more opportunity for the liver to clean the blood. It would be like putting very dirty clothes through the wash two or three times instead of just once. Cleaner blood means a healthier you.

In my opinion, these are some of the reasons why more and more Americans have liver diseases than in any other time in history. We are eating poisons that are killing the liver. Mayonnaise has man-made hydrogenated oil and other ingredients, and was deadly to my liver. Overworking the liver and clogging your body's main filter is dangerous and might be the beginning of disease.

When your liver can no longer metabolize the poisons, thus illness begins. Storing poisons in the body contributes to fatty liver disease and obesity. Your liver is designed to burn fat and NOT store fat. Rejuvenating your liver so it can return to burning fat and NOT storing fat is the goal of this liver cleanse diet.

As your liver becomes healthier and cleans itself, that's when your liver enzyme test results will begin to become normal. If it happened for Mary, it can happen to you with the same mind set. What's that? Eat the suggestions and recipes in this book as if your life depended on it! Because your life does depend on it.

Your body attacks these unknown chemical ingredients in your food as it would any poison – arsenic and all other known poisons. So, for the first week, I want you to only eat the foods I suggest here in this One Week Cleanse for Liver Diseases. After the first week, choose any of the foods from this book.

This is the path that Mary took for her Non-Alcoholic Fatty Liver Disease to be in complete remission. This book contains more recipes than Mary had, so you have a bigger choice of options.

When you fail . . . . you noticed I didn't say, "if you fail." A lifestyle change is difficult. When you fail just pick yourself up, brush yourself off and begin again. It took you eating the mistaken foods for many years to get to where you are now, so – PUH – leeze, don't expect yourself to be perfect in a few hours, days, weeks or even months.

Each step will bring you closer to a healthier you and a healthier liver. As I used to say in my Public Service Announcements on Christian television called, "God's Plan, God's Food,"

The first step for a healthier tomorrow is taken today.

Liver Cleanse – One-Week Plan

- Every day drink one quart of Dr. B's Recipe. (See the Index) Do NOT try to drink half of your body weight for the first or second week. Your body will communicate to you when it is ready for more filtered water without fluoride and unrefined sea salt. Please see the Index, "Dr. B's Recipe" for further details.

- Breakfast Smoothie. (see the recipe in this book) No caffeine drinks – like coffee, tea or soda.

- Add two fresh, RAW fruit snacks. 10:00 a.m. and 3:00 p.m.

- Lunch—large raw salad with EVOO Salad Dressing. (or one of the other dressing choices in this book.)

NOTE:

If you are extremely sick and feel sick to your stomach when you eat the salad dressing, please skip this raw salad for the first three days of your cleanse. Instead, have a lunch of just raw, fresh fruit. Pick whatever fresh fruits that you like or are in season.

- For dinner eat a bowl or two of "Tomato Soup" from the recipe in this book.

- Every night before bed, drink a cup of chamomile tea. (Chamomile tea ingredients: chamomile – that's it.) Yes, you may have a teaspoon of raw honey in it to make it sweet.

- Please no television 30 minutes before bed. Put your feet up and count your blessings. If you can, write your blessings down. Review often.

<u>Tentative schedule</u>—adjust the actual times to meet your personal work schedule and needs. Please don't skip eating any of the foods. If you are stuffed, then eat less. If you are hungry, then eat more. Get full. Feel satisfied.

Please NO caffeine or alcohol drinks during this cleanse. Once you get a normal liver enzyme test, then you can experiment with one caffeine drink per day, but add 24 more ounces of water to counteract the caffeine. More on this later.

Why? Because caffeine constricts the blood vessels of your body. Constricted blood vessels make it very difficult for the body to remove toxins.

Keyword here? EAT. Ya gotta eat to give the correct nutrients to your body so your liver has the tools to repair itself. Don't worry, you won't gain weight. Ninety percent of my students lose weight. Some are worried about eating all of the extra virgin olive oil in the recipes. Don't be. The EVOO will allow your body to remove all of the bad fat you have been eating. EVOO helps you lose weight. Trust me for one week.

- Prepare the crock recipe of tomato soup.

- While you are making your smoothie, please drink one glass of Dr. B's Recipe. (See Index)

- Breakfast Smoothie (you can be creative with this meal, but it must be fresh, raw fruit. See the recipe for more ideas.)

- 10:00 a.m. eat a raw fruit snack. One serving is about one cup. Drink one glass of Dr. B's Recipe. (See Index)

- Lunch—BIG and RAW salad. Nothing cooked or prepared. Use the EVOO Salad dressing in this book or the other dressings in this book. Homemade Flatbread would be wonderful. Drink one glass of Dr. B's Recipe. (See Index)

- 3:00 p.m. snack—more raw fruit. Drink one glass of Dr. B's Recipe. (See Index)

- 6:00 p.m. Dinner—Tomato Soup. Eat until you are full. You may have another raw salad with your soup. A cup of chamomile tea with one teaspoon (or more) of raw honey or Grade A Maple syrup.

- 10:00 p.m. a second cup of chamomile tea and relax with a book or sit and quietly count your blessings.

The reasons why:

Dr. B's Recipe detoxifies your body. Your body is a bag of salt water. Without salt you won't have energy. Unrefined Celtic Sea salt gives energy. Sports drinks have BLEACHED salt that is detrimental to your health, and it contains chemicals that are NOT safe. (See Index: Salt Example)

- Fruit is a perfect detoxification food. The water in the fruit is directly from your Creator. No, you won't gain weight from eating God's perfect sweetness that is contained naturally in the fruit because it is balanced with the essential nutrient we call fiber. No, it is NOT roughage, fiber is a survival nutrient your body needs to make a healthy liver.

- Raw veggies are essential to cleanse you and your liver.

- Soup is one of the easiest foods to digest. Easy digestion gives your liver time to cleanse and repair itself.

- A frequently asked question is: "Why eat so much fruit? Won't I gain weight eating all that sugar? I always assure students that they will NOT gain weight. This is a plan for one week to start your new life style.

The students that ask are usually eating man-made sugars like aspartame. There is a REAL danger of aspartame poisoning. Because aspartame is man-made, your body treats it like a poison and sends it directly to the liver to filter out – thus poisoning your liver.

Eating Aspartame and White, Refined Sugar

causes inflammation of the liver.

People want to cheat their bodies so they buy what they think will fool their body so they won't gain weight. Only problem? These same people will cheat themselves out of their liver's health because eating fake sugar causes inflammation, and inflammation destroys your liver and your health.

If we use history as our judge of a good diet, nowhere in the entire history of the world has there been a culture that has eaten so much refined and man-made sugars as we do today. To match this phenomena, nowhere in the history of the world has there been a culture that has so many health problems.

Dr. Atkins has helped many people lose weight. He writes about Nutra-Sweet and Equal.

"I have taken scores of aspartame-users who seemed to be metabolically resistant to weight loss off this sweetener and observed weight loss to resume."

Dr. Lendon Smith, M.D., author of "Feed yourself right" says,

"In my own practice, I've found that B vitamins help to curb cravings for sugar. And the B's help sour a sweet tooth, too."

How do you get B vitamins? Swallow vitamins? NOOOOOO! Never from a vitamin pill. Eat whole grains. Give up enriched food products and your appetite will be satisfied quicker **and** you will eat the B vitamins that your body craves from your food!

Vitamin Note:

You may have health risks by eating vitamins by themselves. You need the survival ingredients that activate all vitamins, what's that ingredient? Well, it's a secret that vitamin salesmen don't want you to know! That secret is called fiber. Without the essential nutrient of fiber you are wasting your money on single vitamins. Your body processes whole foods that contain the right combination of vitamins made by your Creator. If you believe in evolution, then you evolved with whole foods and NOT a vitamin pill. Please see my website for more information: www.MigrainePhD.com/fiber

You see, fiber is the essential nutrient to activate the vitamins. Are you getting your nutrients with your vitamins? Vitamins are a health myth, but fiber is the essential nutrients secret. Vitamins cannot work unless fiber is present.

That's why fresh fruits and vegetables are so important to the health of human beings. The Creator - God - made it essential that you eat HIS creation in order to maintain your good health. If you believe in evolution, then the same foods that you evolved with must be eaten. Vitamins never evolved with a one-cell animal.

Liver Cleanse – Six-Week Plan

Right around week three, most students "get it" when the light comes on. See adapting your recipes for more information to help you transition to a healthier liver lifestyle. By reading and understanding the concepts, most students become confident enough to start converting their own favorite recipes to encouraging liver function.

Please consider making your own herbal medicine for rejuvenating your liver with Milk Thistle. The National Cancer Institute, and the American Cancer Society says that Milk Thistle may help with liver inflammation. The recipe in this book is for homemade, milk thistle tincture because I do not like any of the store-bought versions on the market today.

This herbal recipe takes six weeks of sitting on your own kitchen counter to create. The recipe is in this book, and a link to the organic milk thistle is on my website. If you start making it soon, you will be ready to add it to your new lifestyle at the end of this six-week liver cleanse.

Taking milk thistle helps to rejuvenate your liver. BUT, a word of CAUTION for Milk Thistle:

Start Slow – about three drops of the tincture every day in a glass of filtered water without fluoride. After a few months, you may want to try seven drops of the tincture in a glass of water. Please do NOT rush.

Why? Because you want to help your body to repair the liver and NOT to force your body to repair. Yes, there is a big difference. Forcing means you want the detoxification to start **NOW**! Nahh. We help the body to work at its own pace and we do not force the body. The body has the wisdom to do what it is supposed to do when given the right tools.

Here's why:

If you take too much Milk Thistle, detoxification that takes place too quickly has uncomfortable side effects. Like what?

- A low-grade headache is how my body reacts.
- Muscle aches.
- Being more tired than usual.
- Nausea, stomach upset, heartburn or a laxative effect.
- ? – I cannot predict the way your body will react. I don't know how sick your liver is at present. Slow and steady wins the race. When in doubt, leave it out. You can always revisit the tincture in a few months. The recipe does not spoil because of the 100-proof vodka you will add. You will be amazed how just changing your food can change your life.

Please, if you have any questions, go to my website to the contact page to get in touch. No charge for one question. I give telephone consultations, too. The first fifteen minutes are free. http://MigrainePhD.com/contact

Liver Cleanse Basic Dietary Goals:

1) Eat at least one fresh raw salad every day. (no meat in salad)

2) Salad dressing made by you and NOT store bought!

3) Eat two snacks every day. A recipe in the book or a fresh fruit snack. No, not dehydrated, not in a can, no salted and not in a package – FRESH or HOMEMADE snacks.

4) Choose two recipes from the recipe section of this book.

5) Eat wild caught fish or sock-eye salmon two times a week or go vegan – no meat no animal products. You pick.

6) Don't forget to drink one quart of Dr. B's Recipe as discussed in the One Week Cleanse every single day.

Week One:

- Mandatory Reading: Partially Hydrogenated Oil #1 Poison. Then give up eating all oils in your diet, but eat EVOO. (extra virgin olive oil)

- Recommended Reading: The "Lazy, Sneaky Cook" Tells All!"

- Don't forget the Basic Dietary Goals listed above.

- Do one of the 21 Ways to Love your Liver in the Addendum of this book.

Week Two:

- Mandatory Reading: Sugar: #2 Poison to your Liver! Then give up eating all man-made sugars.

- Recommended Reading: Liver Cleanse Diet Foundation.

- Don't forget the Basic Dietary Goals listed above.

- Do one of the 21 Ways to Love your Liver in the Addendum of this book.

Week Three:

- Mandatory Reading: Enriched Foods #3 Poison to your Liver! Then give up eating enriched foods.

- Recommended Reading: Healthy Hearsay.

- Don't forget the Basic Dietary Goals.

- Do one of the 21 Ways to Love your Liver in the Addendum of this book.

Week Four:

- Mandatory Reading: Chemicals in Food #4 Poison. Then give up any words on ingredient lists you don't understand or cannot pronounce. Especially – SALT. Food manufacturers use bleached salt. Bleach makes you deceased. Please know that this salt poisons your liver. I consider unrefined Celtic sea salt as a medicine when used as this text suggests.

- Recommended Reading: Food as Medicine.

- Don't forget the Basic Dietary Goals.

- Do one of the 21 Ways to Love your Liver in the Addendum of this book.

Week Five:

- Mandatory Reading: Animal Products # 5 Poison. Give up meat and animal products – except those labeled, "Organic."

- Recommended Reading: Emotional Problems.
- Don't forget following the Basic Dietary Goals.
- Do one of the 21 Ways to Love your Liver in the Addendum of this book.

<u>Week Six:</u>

- Mandatory Reading: Eating Out without being killed. Follow the rules in this chapter when you eat out OR stop eating out until your liver enzyme test is normal.
- Don't forget the Basic Dietary Goals.
- Recommended Reading: Myths & Weight Loss.
- Do one of the 21 Ways to Love your Liver in the Addendum of this book.

These suggestions are NOT a life sentence. Think of this as a 6-week experiment. You may want to stop the experiment when you receive a good liver test from your doctor. Why should you wait until then? Because you need to have an established base line to know what it feels like to feel good again.

Most of my students have forgotten. This way you will know an old food is wrong for you IF you feel bad after eating it. Use your thoughts to go back in time about 48 hours and to think of what you added to your diet that changed how you feel.

The "Lazy, Sneaky Cook" Tells All!

At my house, dinner is ready when the fire alarm goes off. Yes, I have had a fire or two in my kitchen. Here is a story I don't tell everyone, but since you are joining the ranks of a health NUT – just like me - here goes:

Real Life Story:

One evening at 5:00 p.m., I met my family for dinner on the front porch. Why was I sitting on the front porch? The house was full of smoke. My frying pan had gone up in a blaze! If it were not for my trusty fire extinguisher, I might have lost the house. There were big heat blisters on my stove's exhaust hood where the flames were leaping from the fry pan. I had to repaint the kitchen because of the smoke stains on the walls.

Please do not expect to find any gourmet meals in the Recipe Plan for entertaining and "ahhh-ing" your guests. The meals are just fast, lazy, and sneaky cooking. Why sneaky? Well, that is the next important fact you should know and practice. Puh-leeze!

Do not tell anyone this food is healthy for him or her!

Right now, please raise your right hand and repeat after me, "I promise not to tell anyone this food is healthy!"

If you tell friends and family this food is healthy, they will spit the food out before they taste it. It will be our little secret. Okay? If you are unable to contain your sneaky, little self, you can confess. HOWEVER, only tell everyone <u>after</u> they have finished eating. Promise? Ya gotta promise!

I call my kitchen the "Test Kitchen" because I try to create easy meals that do not require special ingredients or hard-to-find foods. If I cannot find the ingredient at my local grocery, I skip it. <u>A few of the Test Kitchen's priorities:</u>

- Easy preparation.

- No dairy products.

- No prepared, processed foods. (Additives subtract from your health.)

- No store-bought condiments. (Example: Mayo, ketchup, mustard, etc. because of the "poisons" in their ingredient lists.)

- No fake sugar or processed anything.

- No foods that are enriched.

- No white, refined sugar.

- Organic meats eaten a MAXIMUM of two times a day. (Serving size should be about the size of a deck of playing cards.)

That may sound like radical guidelines, but I will discuss the reasons why I have established these priorities. Most recipe books use dairy as the key ingredient to rich-tasting meals. Nope, dairy is not part of this Recipe Plan. There are too many hormones injected into the animals and man-made processed foods that contain chemicals. Even simple food coloring is simply deadly to your liver.

The experts tell us that most homemakers have about 12 recipes that they normally use every day. That is not a lot of recipes. My three lazy favorites?

1. Red Beans and Rice
2. Chicken and Yellow Rice
3. Potato/Tomato Soup

The hardest part of eating without additives will be foraging for your food—I mean shopping for your food. Our ancestors had to search for food, and it is no different today. Searching to find a salad dressing without MSG (monosodium glutamate) or propylene glycol is sometimes difficult at your local grocery store. Ask my student, Jay, who spent 45 minutes searching every salad dressing in the grocery store for a "legal" one. Did he find one? Nope. Now, Jay makes his own salad dressing from the recipe in this book. He's happy.

Many cookbooks call for Dijon mustard and other prepared foods to add extra "flavor" to their recipes quickly. What is the flavor? Chemicals. You can't identify what taste is in the processed foods because the foods just taste good. You don't taste basil. You don't taste oregano. You just taste good. That is a sure sign you are eating chemicals that activate the pleasure center of your brain.

Condiments stay in your refrigerator for months, even years, and never taste bad. How? Think about it. You probably have shoes in your closet that do not last as long as the condiments last in your refrigerator. The answer is simple--these foods are not food. They are just chemicals.

Advertisers boast low cholesterol on their food labels, but what they don't tell us is their products usually contain partially hydrogenated oil or trans-fatty acids that raise cholesterol levels. This is a bad fat. Remember, Food Manufacturers are interested in their bottom line, and not in your life line. Healthy customers have no value to them – just paying customers.

Today, most people think that enriched flour products are good for them. In reality, enriched flour is not food. That is right-- enriched flour has zero food value and will add to your unbalanced health.

All-purpose flour has no purpose.

The first two weeks on this Plan will be the hardest because you must learn to read food labels and develop a new routine. Hang in there. It is worth it! This works.

Most people who see the Recipe Plan think that I love to cook. Hold it, brother! I'm the sneaky, <u>LAZY</u> cook. Anyone who is lazy, would prefer to go to a restaurant, and let THEM do the cooking, the cleaning and the serving for you. It's fast, it's cheap and it's very lazy.

BUT, when I eat out, I get sick the next day. I feel heavy, bloated, no energy and sometimes I would get a migraine headache. I have guidelines in this book how to eat out without being killed, and yes that will help, but there is always a risk of becoming sick when my two little hands don't cook my meal.

The recipes contained in this Recipe Plan are the ones that I use every day. They are easy and fast, but never as fast as going to a restaurant. The way I look at it? Going to a restaurant may be quicker and easier – for the moment, BUT if I add all the time I spend feeling bad and the time I'm out of commission being sick, then eating out takes much more time and more pain.

In this recipe book, when you see "one can of beans," puh-leeze, any can of beans will do. Don't sweat it. White beans, navy beans, pinto beans, BUT the ingredients can only say: "beans" That's it. The ingredient label cannot say, "prepared beans." I don't know what that is. Prepared how?

Celtic Sea salt is a life-giving nutrient and necessary for a healthy life. Real Salt – a brand name salt should be avoided. I have eaten it and it gives me a headache. All Table Salt is deadly because it is bleached, and is NOT good for your liver.

The cheapest salt available may be iodized salt. Iodized salt contains aluminum in it and should be avoided because absorption of aluminum by the brain may be linked to Alzheimer's Disease.

When you see "spice" on an ingredient list, it may be a chemical additive called monosodium glutamate. Monosodium glutamate or MSG kills brain cells, and will give me a migraine headache. MSG poisons your liver.

Broth from a can or jar may have more chemicals under the disguise of "broth." The FDA allows Food Manufacturers to be vague in their labeling of foods. Using different types of beans in the recipes will give a little difference in texture and taste. The best beans to eat are the beans you make with your two little hands. Yes, there is a crock recipe in this book.

Most of the time, I use homemade white beans. Be flexible. I home-can my beans for control over the container. Canned beans are in a can. Duh? But, my homemade canned beans are in glass.

Tin from the can will leech into your food along with the BPA plastic to line most canned goods. Glass does NOT leech into your food. A much better choice. When I cook with my two little hands, I control how many migraines I have. How many migraines do I have? Zero! This same attitude will encourage your liver to heal.

Microwave Warning:

According to Andrew Weil, M.D., you should avoid using the microwave for longer than one minute on, wait one minute and then use one more minute. That's it. Or you may disrupt the food's molecular structure. My personal preference? I do NOT own or use a microwave in my kitchen - ever.

Use the best meat available to you. When we are out of town and camping, and I am forced to shop locally, I search for hormone-free meat. Like grass-fed beef. If it isn't available, I skip it.

It will take time to get a routine for finding new ways to grocery shop. Be fussy, and be prepared to walk out of the store if it doesn't have what you need. Tell the manager on your way out. Real Life Story:

I told one manager: "The grocery store across the street has free-range chicken eggs." I thanked him for his time and walked out of his store.

One month later when I went to that same grocery store, they stocked free-range chicken eggs. It worked. Hormone-free turkeys are usually available around the holidays from your local health food store. Free-range chickens are plentiful in most supermarkets. Tyson advertises in the media and boasting their chickens are free to roam and they don't use hormones. Based on the price – cheap? I would say they are bending the advertising rules in some way.

Because most of our livestock in the United States are pumped with drugs, you won't find any dairy from cows in my recipes. Why? I cannot find good milk products from a sick cow. The organic versions of milk and other dairy products are not as safe as you may think. Try to avoid all dairy. This book will show you how.

I do NOT suggest drinking soy products of any kind. Soy is good for anyone needing estrogen. I have zero students that need estrogen. Body fat in your body makes estrogen. Plus, soymilk is hard to find without additives, too. I have even found "flavoring" in soymilk from health food stores. Flavorings is another name for "MSG." Deadly to the health of your liver.

Two soy recipes I had from previous cookbooks have been dropped for this reason. My only alternative for grated cheese is to use grated goat's or sheep's milk cheese. Ask your grocer and keep searching. Both Costco and SAMS sell this type of cheese. This is NOT food as medicine, but okay food.

Okay food can only be twenty percent of your total eating when your liver enzyme test comes back normal. Until then, use the amounts I suggest in the recipes or skip using the sheep's milk cheese for now.

A lifestyle cannot be based on eating okay food – especially for someone who wants to improve the health of their liver. Used sparingly as a sprinkling will work, but it can also be skipped.

Beware of buying soy products because Food Manufacturers love to jump on the "Healthy Hearsay" bandwagon. Here's another example of something that should be good for you, or is it? Soy meat. Vegetarians can add "meat-like" protein to their diet and not eat meat. Here is the problem – too much man-made chemicals added to the soy meat. Avoid it. Here's why.

What Food Manufacturers do to the innocent little soybean is a crime. The soybean proteins are dissolved into alkali, and then put into an acid bath. This "poison" is now tasteless and odorless. No problem for Food Manufacturers: they add artificial flavor, color, and artificial or natural flavoring and tah dah! Poison! I mean, "soy meat?" This "poison" can be camouflaged into looking like chicken, ham, fish, hot dogs, hamburger--you name it. Most important - don't eat it.

Celtic Sea salt is necessary for good health. These recipes are geared for my taste buds. Once you cook a recipe, you can improve upon it so it matches the taste buds of your family. Celtic sea salt in recipes is needed for good health. Your brain is 85 percent salt water and needs salt to function and think.

Water Requirement:

Please know that most Americans are dehydrated and need to drink more water in their diets. If you drink one caffeine drink per day, it robs your body of three times its water amount. Yes, you can drink caffeine, but you MUST add 24 ounces more water to replace the water robbed from your body.

Pre-heating oven:

I RARELY preheat my oven in any of my recipes. One Youtube viewer ranted and raved that "nobody cooks that way!" No problem, I am NOT a trained chef nor do I profess to be well coordinated in the kitchen. In fact, I am rather awkward when it comes to me being around a hot oven. How do I avoid this dilemma? I do NOT preheat my oven. Sorry to disappoint all you chefs out there.

Is Pizza Delivery okay food?

I'm often asked, "Is pizza healthy?" I always respond, "Who made it?" Yes, the pizza recipe in this book is healthy. I can't eat pizza delivery or pizza in the frozen food section because it makes me feel sick. Food Manufacturers use "Spice" in their processed—whatever it is—food? Here are three reasons why pizza delivery is "Don't touch it" food:

1. The crust is enriched flour. Enriched flour is not food—it's paste. It clogs my plumbing, makes me feel bloated, and the "cravings" for more pizza than I should probably eat is overwhelming.

2. Pepperoni, bacon or sausage will give me a migraine. The chemical called, "nitrates" is in all processed meat in the United States. Why? Because "they" (I imagine it's the Food Manufacturers and the FDA) are positive that consumers will eat processed meat raw and not cook it. Not healthy. So, "they" are protecting us dummies. Don't worry, vitamin C is added and may stop the nitrates from causing cancer in humans. Does it? I dunno. I still get a migraine. That means nitrates attack your liver.

The American Cancer Society says that it takes 20 years to get cancer. 20 years of eating "poison" in your diet. "Poison" gives me a migraine, others get cancer or liver disease.

3. Sauce. When pizza restaurants offer pizza delivered to your house for $5.99, they gotta have a profit! Right? The sauce is most likely the place to build in profit. They add chemicals which will preserve their sauce. I

mean, the pizza in this cookbook probably "costs" $5.99 to make yourself. These chemicals are not something available for consumers to cook with in our own kitchens. Like propylene glycol for a cheaper sweetener than sugar for the sauce. It's a kind of antifreeze. What do they think we are—cars? No, they want profits.

Liver Cleanse Diet Foundation

The foundation of this way of eating is based on the concept that feeling better comes from medicine from the farm and not from the pharmacy. When I was suffering from migraine headaches, I went to see my trusty M.D. He did exactly what he was taught to do in medical school:

- he examined.
- he diagnosed.
- he wrote a prescription to help with the symptom--pain.
- he educated me how to use the medication.

In his mind, his job was performed the exact way he was taught in medical school. He told me that the medication would enlarge the blood vessels in my head. I was petrified. He didn't have an answer to my question, "Why am I having these headaches?"

One of the answers to my migraines was so simple, it almost stumped me. It was the "poison" in my food. I eliminated the "poison," and the migraines disappeared. What "poison?" Go to your cupboard and look at a can or box of something. Sure, do it now. I'll wait here.

Read the ingredients. No, not the front of the label--the back. The "poison" is all those words you cannot pronounce. You need to be a chemist to know what the words mean or how to pronounce them. I eliminated all of that "poison," and now my migraines are in total remission.

This is the basis of why Mary's fatty liver disease went into remission. I have shared my "migraine diet" with students, and they, too, have had success reducing their migraines and other diseases.

Two or three years after my discovery of this diet, I learned about a medical doctor who made a similar discovery for his migraine headaches--Max Gerson, M.D.

When Max Gerson was a young medical student, he had migraines. When he asked his medical school professors how to help the headaches, they gave him no hope for a cure. They simply told him, "Learn to live with them and when you are 50 they should decrease."

WHAT? The young medical student began searching to find his cure. He heard about a woman in Italy who was controlling her migraines with diet, and he decided to try to do the same.

Through trial and error, Max Gerson discovered what he eventually called his, "migraine diet." It worked. When Max Gerson became a medical doctor, he shared his discovery with his patients who had migraines. They, too, announced pain relief.

One patient reported that he had been healed from tuberculosis. Dr. Gerson was shocked. He offered to treat others with tuberculosis free of charge in an effort to see if they could be healed with his "migraine diet." Other patients with tuberculosis were healed.

Later, Dr. Gerson adapted his migraine diet and used it to cure cancer. Oh, by the way, Dr. Gerson discovered his migraine diet in the early 1930's. His cancer clinic is still operating today in Mexico. I have visited his clinic in Tijuana, Mexico. Why did a U.S. doctor move his clinic to Mexico? Because in the U.S. it is illegal to cure cancer with diet. There are ONLY three acceptable ways to cure cancer in America according to the American Medical Association:

- Surgery
- Chemo therapy
- Radiation therapy

Dr. Gerson's dietary methods did not comply. His medical license was revoked, and he brought his life-saving treatment to Mexico.

I am honored that my discovery that food is medicine is in good company with Dr. Max Gerson. However, Solomon was right, "There's nothing new under the sun." Seventy-five years ago Dr. Gerson healed cancer with food and two thousand years ago Hippocrates said, "Let your medicine be your food. Let your food be your medicine." Hippocrates is considered by many to be the "Father of Medicine." He taught this "Food-as-Medicine" concept to his students and practiced it with his patients.

Today. this same concept of food as medicine causes people who have liver diseases to go into remission. The body reacts in different ways to the same poisons. That is the reason why heredity plays such a large part in main-stream medicine. Heredity determines WHERE you have cancer and not IF you get cancer.

I had migraines because both my father and my mother suffered with them. My daughter has migraines because of me and my parents passing the weak trait along to her. Heredity means the "weak" part of a family's history predisposes me to the same diseases.

Now, the good news, I changed the way I eat, and my daughter followed my footsteps and neither of us suffers with migraines anymore. If I cook like my parents, I will have the same diseases of my parents.

This will happen for you. The liver problems will disappear when you start following the same concepts in this book. Yes, Dr. Max's diet cured cancer patients. His text, "A Cancer Therapy," documents 50 cases that his adapted migraine diet cured.

One acquaintance of mine hopes she has inherited the good genes from her mother. Her mother lived past 100 years of age, had lots of energy and full intelligence. She died in an unfortunate accident while living in a retirement home. Her mother was raised on a farm, ate home-canned food from her garden, and rarely ate food prepared by eating out.

On the other hand, my acquaintance eats out often, likes prepared food, and doesn't like to cook. She got cancer at 60 years old, and probably feels she did not inherit her mom's genes. Unfortunately, my research proves that health is earned by eating God's foods every day to invest in good health for your future.

We are not cursed by God giving us the wrong set of parents with the wrong set of genes. If my acquaintance had followed in her Mom's eating footsteps, chances are good she never would have gotten cancer.

My friend decided to do chemo therapy, and not take my suggestions in this book. She took chemo therapy and traded her cancer for dementia. At 65, she was admitted to a nursing home and spent the rest of her life living there not recognizing her family.

Many Americans are sick, and medical science does not know why. Human nature needs to blame something. Consequently, blaming illness on heredity seems to be common practice. My research demonstrates that the only thing we inherit are the "genetic weaknesses towards getting the disease"--not the actual disease.

In addition, to the inheriting genetic weakness, we inherit the cookbooks from our parents. The cookbooks are an important link to our lifestyle of eating habits. Diet is an important link to disease and is – in my opinion - the cause for most illness.

Change the diet; change the chance to develop disease. Health is earned and NOT found in a prescription drug or surgery.

According to the New York Times 2000 Almanac, in 1960 the national expenditure for health care in the United States was $16.9 billion and rose to $1,092 billion in 1997. That means we are spending 64 times more for health care in 1997 than we did in 1960! Shocking!

From 1990 to 1997, health care expenditures almost doubled. Folks, we are spending more than a trillion dollars on health care. Yes, costs are up, but Americans are sicker than in any other time in history. If there were an award for the sickest nation on earth, Americans would take the trophy without much competition. What is a contributing cause to increased illness?

Today, Americans rely on doctors to "fix" them up rather than taking responsibility for their own health. It's like the farmer's tractor that was stalling out. The mechanic replaced the carburetor, but never asked the farmer what kind of fuel he was giving the tractor. The mechanic makes money for replacing the carburetor, and not for selling the farmer fuel.

In a short time, the tractor had the same stalling out problem, because the farmer was using old, watered-down fuel from the barn in his tractor. The mechanic was happy to repair the tractor a second time.

To relate our farmer and his tractor story to our body, the "ingredient list" tells you what kind of "fuel" you are "using" into your body. Putting on a new carburetor would be like a person having bypass surgery. The surgery is a "fix" for eating processed foods that have been "watered down" with "poison." (Poison would be preservatives and chemicals in the food.)

If the farmer had changed the fuel for his tractor, he could have avoided the second new carburetor repair. If liver cancer patients would change their diet, they might avoid the need for a liver transplant.

Never has any culture's food been so tampered with than it is today. Just try to read the list of ingredients on any package you have in your pantry. I say, "try to" because Food Manufacturers use color combinations that make reading this information unreadable. I am talking about a package with yellow printed on an orange background. The label is not meant for reading. The label is meant to comply with the rules of the FDA. (Federal Drug Administration)

Indeed, you would need a degree as a food chemist to understand the information printed there. Think about that. You are eating chemicals in your food that weren't invented or thought of when your grandmother or grandfather was young. Is there any wonder why our generation is sicker and has higher health care costs than any generation before us?

"We don't know what these chemicals do to the human body."
Ben F. Feingold, M.D.

Yes, Dr. Feingold, you are right. Illness is skyrocketing because no one is doing any research on the impact these food additives and other chemicals have on physical or emotional health. From depression, diabetes, heart palpitations to liver disease – my students have demonstrated to me that processed food contributes to illness. It is difficult to pinpoint exactly what these chemicals do to our health because different people have different health symptoms from eating the same chemical in their food.
Real Life Story:

I went on a double date with some friends. After our bike ride, we went to eat at a fancy restaurant for lunch. There was a lunch special, so we all had the same meal for lunch.

After lunch, my girlfriend did not make it home before she had to rush to the bathroom with horrible cramps. My date told me he had to take a nap on the couch when he got home. He rarely naps. At 3:00 a.m., I woke up with a horrible migraine, and nothing happened to my girlfriend's husband. We all ate the same chemicals at lunch, but each person had a different set of symptoms.

Why is no one doing the research to find out if there is a connection between the additives we eat and disease? Because no one wants to know. Food manufacturing is much too profitable. Kraft claimed $87 billion as part of their processed food market share of profit in 2001!

In great-grandmother's day, the kitchen was the meeting place, a place of fellowship and coming together to make the family meal. "Together" is the keyword. The family made the meal together because it was a lot of hard work. It still is.

Trying to involve children to make and prepare their own food will help them own this way of eating and save them from health problems when they grow up.

* Picky eaters will usually eat what they made.
* Owning what they eat because they made a choice in choosing the food.
* Learning that food making is important to you, then it will become important to them.
* Bonds you and the child together doing an activity that doesn't entertain them. They are providing their own entertainment.
* Starts a dialog with the child to learn what foods are healthy and what foods are NOT healthy. When the child is absent from you, they have a better understanding of what they should or should NOT eat.

As the Bible verse says,

> *"Train up a child in the way he should go,*
>
> *and when he is old he will not depart from it."*

* A child is NOT born knowing how much sweet tastes good. Do NOT add sugar to your child's food. Don't pass your bad habits onto your child.

* Sweet is natural for all children to want some. Keep the sweets natural – like fresh fruits or adding raw honey. Keeping their diet simple and without white, refined sugar is a smart goal. The longer you wait to share their first, store– bought ice cream the longer their taste buds will develop to prefer natural sweetness to un-natural sweet desserts.

"SAT scores are the lowest in 50 years."
Joseph Beasley, M.D.

Kids are regularly given prescription medication for ADD & ADHD that were unknown diseases in the 40's and 50's. Our teachers are the best trained anywhere on the planet, but other cultures score better than American kids. Why?

"An artificial food color, such as the chemical tartrazine- Food, Drug & Cosmetic (FD &C) Yellow #5 –
can have within the human body the same manner as
a "drug" used for medication."
Ben F. Feingold, M.D.

We drug our children with food additives in their food that makes it necessary to NEED drugs like Prozac. SAT scores are down because of the processed food that our kids eat every day. The "lunchable-type" food, chips, drive-thru meals, and other non-food our children eat regularly make them hyper.

Lower test scores are not because of the teaching techniques. Other cultures don't have better teachers than in the U.S. Other cultures just don't have as much processed food as the U.S. They don't have fast food on every corner, and they don't want it. They know that food is foundational to their children's ability to learn. Americans? They gotta have a easy lifestyle and cheap food.

For the first time in the history of the world, we have obese children. Yes, I agree that children need physical education, but food is the foundation of your life and your child's life.

Nutra-babble is confusing consumers so much that we don't know what is true and what is false. I call this "Healthy Hearsay." There is so much nonsense talk about "getting your protein," to the crazy concept that you cannot mix one food with another food because the human stomach cannot digest a mixture.

In reality, people have digestion problems because of the chemicals in food and their lack of drinking enough filtered water without fluoride. God's creation is "fearfully and wonderfully made." The human stomach has hydrochloric acid and can dissolve itself within a few hours if its self-protecting mucus lining were broken.

One minute Healthy Hearsay tells you that eating margarine is fine and the next minute eat butter. Wait a few months and they will change their minds - again. None of it is true. Do you hear me?

NONE OF IT IS TRUE!

Here are the only two things to be concerned about for good nutrition:

1) If it's God's whole food, it's good for your health. (This food does NOT have a label.)

2) If it's processed, man-made food, it's bad for your health. (This food has a label.)

Two categories of food. Simple. Too simple - right? God wants His kids healthy. So, God made it simple!

The hardest part of this Liver Cleanse Plan will be changing the way you think about food. This Liver Cleanse Plan does not take any will power - it just takes a lot of plan power.

No, there's no need to worry about food combining. God's nutrition is easy. If God made it and man has not processed it, you can eat it.

Yes, you can eat organic meat, but in much smaller quantities than most Americans normally eat meat. Meat in your diet should account for 15 percent at any one meal. Why limit meat? Unless you are a farmer eating your own animals that you raised, you must limit meat. Food Manufacturers **CANNOT** be trusted.

Meat should be a sprinkling on your food or a serving about the size of a deck of cards on your plate. In 2015, I became a vegan. I am not suggesting you become a vegan that is your choice. My book, "The Virgin Vegan's Secret Walmart Recipes" has beginning recipes without meat and animal products will show you how. These recipes are liver friendly.

For the scope of this book in order for you to have a normal liver enzyme test result, I am suggesting that you eat at least one meatless meal each day. How? Eat a daily, very large, raw salad is the foundation of this Liver Cleanse Plan. God dictated to Moses which meats were acceptable to eat. See Leviticus 11.

Briefly:

- No pork
- No Shrimp
- No Catfish
- No Scallops
- No Lobster

As a guess, maybe God says to stay away from these animals because they are all scavengers. In the Bible, God calls this food, "FILTH." Yikes! You can make this decision for yourself. For me, I'm not eatin' any filth.

Food Manufacturers CANNOT be trusted when raising scavenger varieties of animals because of the animals' nature is to eat filth. What they eat may be harmful to humans.

<u>Concentrate on the positives.</u>

There are so many different types of good food; I prefer to concentrate on what I can eat instead of what food limitations that are placed on food by anyone.

You decide for your body. Whatever type of meat you decide to eat, please eat the non-hormone variety of that meat. Next, let's discuss "What is healthy."

Healthy Hearsay

Most people never take a formal class about what to eat and to learn "What is healthy." This is a tragedy because people in America rely on Healthy Hearsay for the foundation of their healthy eating habits.

Sidney MacDonald Baker, M.D. tells a story of one of his patients who decided he wanted to get "healthy." He was drinking six beers every night after work and all his friends told him that beer was not healthy.

In an effort to do what his friends told him was "healthy," he made a dietary change. What did he decide to do? He switched to drinking six diet colas every night. In my opinion, aspartame is deadly and not a better choice to drinking beers. The proof?

In three months, he was rushed to the emergency room because he was having uncontrollable seizures! What's healthy? This man was a victim of Healthy Hearsay! Diet drinks with fake sugar kills brain cells.

What is Healthy?

It depends on who you ask.

If you ask a vitamin salesperson at a health food store, you will probably get a list of vitamins you need to eat. If you ask a medical doctor, you may get a prescription. If you ask a personal trainer, you will be shown how to exercise efficiently.

The list goes on and on as to the various answers to what you thought was a simple question. What is healthy is a simple question with lots of different answers – depending on who you ask.

It's like asking a used car sales clerk if he thinks you should trade your car or not. You will most likely get a biased answer. YES, trade your car, and buy a car from him.

<u>Healthy Hearsay - Low Fat</u>

Since the 1970's, low fat food products have become very popular. The problem is that Healthy Hearsay says, eat "no fat" or eat "low fat" if you want to become thin." There is low-fat ice cream, yogurt, chips, salad dressing, cookies, cheese, and frozen entrées, BUT Americans are still becoming obese. Why?

"Low fat" is a big fat lie!"

Dr. Dean Ornish says don't eat fat, and Dr. Robert Atkins says eat nothing but fat. (The Zone and Sugar Busters, too.) Duh? Healthy Hearsay has everyone confused. Who is right? Neither.

"Very low-fat diets may even deprive the body of important nutrients that defend against heart disease and cancer,"

Kevin Vigilante, M.D.

Low fat is dangerous because good fat versus bad fat is never mentioned. Your liver's number one enemy? BAD fat. High fat is dangerous because a high-meat diet is very hard for the body to filter - - especially the kidneys.

Real Life Story::

A friend of mine wanted to lose weight before her wedding. She decided to try the Adkins Diet – it was popular at that time. What happened? Apparently, she did not have strong kidneys to keep up with the high demand of digesting all the meat and had a highly-concentrated waste that caused her to be rushed to the emergency room for kidney failure.

This Liver Cleanse Plan suggests you eat lots of fat in the food of EVOO, that's extra virgin olive oil. That is just one of the reasons why anyone who has eaten this Plan loses weight. Eating good fat detoxifies the liver. A healthy liver helps you live.

Good fat helps you lose weight.

Healthy Hearsay - Natural

Our government has NOT given a clear definition to the word "natural" to Food Manufacturers. Consequently, "natural" is totally without meaning. If you see that word, don't believe it. Put the package down and RUN!

My definition of natural would be a comb carved of wood. Un-natural or man-made would be a plastic comb because plastic is not found anywhere in nature. Oil pressed from olives without chemicals or detergents would be called natural.

Oil that has been hydrogenated and molecularly changed like soybean oil would be called man-made. This would be logical, right? It may be logical to me, but not to Food Manufacturers.

Food Manufacturers twist logic to meet their needs. What are their needs? To make money selling their "poison." I have seen potato chip labels that say, "ALL NATURAL" and the ingredient list contains man-made, molecularly-changed oil called, "partially hydrogenated oil." Duh? How? Remember, there isn't a clear definition to "natural." They can say whatever they want.

On the other hand, how about popular parmesan cheese that states on the label, "100% Grated Parmesan Cheese," and it has chemicals listed in the ingredient list. How? I decided to call the 1-800 number on this product. Here's what the "el wise ones" told me: "The product is 100% "grated" not 100% all parmesan cheese." Hmmmmm.

One more "natural" that isn't natural. What? Coffee that is "naturally decaffeinated." Why? Because Food Manufacturers use too many chemicals to remove the caffeine. If you call the 1-800 number, you get a run-around about exactly "how" they take out the caffeine.

Think about this: Caffeine is "natural" to the coffee bean. If you take out the caffeine from the coffee, it is no longer "natural." Therefore, how can decaffeinated coffee be naturally decaffeinated using water? Ain't no way!

Plus, removing all the caffeine is NOT possible. They can only remove 70 percent of the caffeine. That's close enough for the FDA to look the other way. Decaf may NOT be part of your menu if you want a healthy liver. Give it up until you get a good liver enzyme test.

Healthy Hearsay - Organic

Another Healthy Hearsay is the word "organic." Many people think that if the label says, "organic," it has a special Healthy Hearsay blessing on it. (Organic for buying meat is the only exception.) Nope. I have seen some scary ingredients on a label of soymilk while in the health food store. Folks, just 'cause it's in the health food store does not make it healthy! If I stand in the barn and neigh like a horse, it doesn't make me a horse, right?

Healthy Hearsay is dangerous. Why? Because most Healthy Hearsay is written by advertisers who want to sell their "stuff." How do you know when an advertiser is lying? Answer: When their lips are moving, of course.

Read ingredient lists - it's our only defense. The best food to eat does NOT have an ingredient label.

A definition of organic might be not using chemicals to fertilize the ground or to keep bugs off. (pesticides) Farmers would rotate their crop by giving the land a rest period. I dunno. I'm a city kid. If these were the guidelines, when does the ground become organic?

Ask yourself, "Self, is the ground organic in one week of no chemicals? Does the land have to be sterilized first? Can farmers use a special seed that has been "genetically engineered" to repel bugs?" Think about that one for a moment. If bugs, the lowest life form, doesn't want to eat your food and stays away from veggies with this type of seed, is it still food?

Since I am not a farmer, I am unsure about the list of farming variables. Organic is NOT magic food. If Food Manufacturers add chemicals to your "organic" food, it is still bad for your liver. One student told me that she knew she was eating healthy because her food said "organic." She thought if she bought all organic food at the health food store, she was eating healthy. Not so.

I found applesauce in a grocery store that was "natural" and it cost $1.47. A similar applesauce in a similar jar but at the health food store was $3.79. Organic carries a heavy price tag. But, is one product better than the other? Both had similar ingredients that said: apples. The health food store said "organic apples" and the regular grocery store said, "apples."

A farmer's market or produce stand is my choice for fresh fruit and vegetables based on the information I have today.

Healthy Hearsay – Protein:

In America, athletes and most health nuts are overly concerned about getting their protein. No, I'm not talking about the protein you can get from beans, nuts, seeds, potatoes, and whole grains. I am talking about MEAT protein.

Okay, let's think about this from another point of view: Here's an example of a person needing a lot of protein to make muscle. A newborn baby is born at about seven pounds and maybe twenty-one inches long.

In the first year of life, that infant transforms from a limp, sleeps-all-the time infant to a little kid who may be running around the house grabbing anything that is not nailed down. This infant almost doubles in weight and height, and muscles that were not strong enough to hold his head up-to now climbing and jumping on the sofa. How much protein does a baby eat? Lots of protein, huh? Arrrgh! MEAT!

Nope. Mother's milk, the best food for babies (even doctors and scientists agree on that) is 1.8 percent protein. Folks, a baked potato has 1.8 percent protein! Meat is NOT as necessary as many Food Manufacturers want us to believe!

More evidence of this inaccuracy is the value body builders place on high protein shakes and protein bars. It is nothing but hype to line their pockets with your money. Hype that loads up the liver with chemicals and poisons!

Think of the strongest animal you know. Did you say elephant? Gorilla? How much meat protein do they eat? Zero! They eat green veggies, not meat. Try arm wrestling with a gorilla and tell me how you do.

Healthy Hearsay - Exercise

Changing your diet will give you the desire to exercise because you will have more energy. If you have friends that are part of the "get-healthy-through-exercise" crowd, but they ignore

their diet because of the false belief that exercise makes them immune to heart disease, read on for another point of view!
Real Life Story:

Author Jim Fixx trained as a marathoner since the age of 15. He was lean at 6 feet 1 inch and 150 pounds. He looked healthy and his slow pulse and low blood pressure proved he was healthy, or was he? He did the right things to be healthy: he was a nonsmoker, limited alcohol and was an athlete of 25 years.

Jim Fixx was VERY knowledgeable about his love for running. He wrote three successful books on running. Two of the books became favorite references for runners, and one became a best seller in all of publishing history. He competed and finished six Boston marathons, won the Connecticut 10,000-meter championship in his age category, and ran the equivalent of once around the equator. This man ran ten miles every day. Does he sound like a successful athlete to you? Yup, you bet. I'm very impressed.

One problem--Jim's diet. Nathan Pritikin in his book, <u>Nathan Pritikin Diet for Runners</u> writes:

"In July, 1976, Jim Fixx was interviewed by the London Daily Mail. Fixx described with some glee-and a certain arrogance--his breakfast that morning of fried eggs, sausage, bacon, buttered white toast and coffee with cream. Jim Fixx was quoted as saying, "If you run, you can participate fully in the ways of our civilization and get away with it."

Later in the same year, Jim Fixx ran three hours over hilly terrain in preparation for his next marathon. Jim "believed" that exercise made him immune to heart disease. The following day in Oakland, California, Jim Fixx died of a massive heart attack while running at the age of 42.

Jim Fixx exercised for health, but he died for diet.

Don't bet your life on Healthy Hearsay. By-pass surgery is sometimes thought to be an easy fix to eating "the ways of our civilization." (By the way, 452,000 bypass operations were performed in the U.S. in 1996) Jim Fixx didn't get a chance to fix his way of eating with this surgery. For your friends thinking about letting their doctor "fix them" with by-pass surgery, think again. By-pass surgery has side effects, too.

In February, 2001, a Duke University study shocked the multi-billion-dollar heart bypass industry with a stunning report that was based on 261 patients who had bypass surgery at Duke from 1989 to 1993. The study relied on mental tests done before surgery and then taking the same test at six weeks, six months, and five years AFTER by-pass surgery.

- The patients' average age was 61, with a range of 50 to 71.
- Patients were considered to have declined mentally if their test performance at five years was at least 20 percent lower than their score before surgery.

The results: The drop in scores was more than two-to-three times the mental decline found in 5,888 Medicare patients who did not have bypass surgery and whose cognitive abilities were followed for five years in a separate study.

The National Health Federation writes:

"Some 42 percent of 261 patients who had bypass surgery at Duke between 1989 and 1993 showed evidence of significant declines on tests of mental ability - probably from damage to the their brain during the by-pass procedure."

Scary? That's almost half - there's more.

Nathan Pritikin writes,

"You may not be aware that of all people who undergo coronary bypass surgery, 10-to-20 percent suffer complete blockage of their bypasses within the first year."

If you have heart disease, or have a family history that indicates you have a weakness towards heart disease, please pay close attention to the section titled, "Poison - Animal Products," for another theory. This new theory indicates that heart disease is a hormonal disorder and not related to the good and bad cholesterol theory of mainstream medical science teaches today. Stay tuned-- more about that theory later.

Food as Medicine

This is a VERY important concept to understand. The concept is simple. In fact, it may be too simple, if that is possible. I have had students that know too much. I mean, they knew more Healthy Hearsay than was good for their own health.

However, what they "knew" is what many, many people have told them or, worse yet, information that was written by advertisers. When you read an article in a magazine that is boasting a "miracle" juice and all its amazing powers, it is <u>no coincidence</u> the same juice has an advertisement in the same magazine--that month, last month or next month.

Biased information is dangerous information. Just 'cause you read it in a magazine, does NOT make it true. Eating Food as Medicine does <u>not</u> mean you should stop taking your prescription medication from your physician! Puh-leeze! Getting off prescription medication is a serious matter for you to discuss with the doctor who prescribed the medication for you. Not me. Not this book.

If you follow the eating guidelines in this book, your doctor's examination will naturally reveal he can take you off medication. Your doctor was trained how to:

* read test results to prescribe medication
* read test results to stop medication

You must start thinking of food as your medicine and investing time to make your own food so you can help your liver have the right tools to become healthy.

- You are not just eating a meal – you are eating medicine.

- Food is no longer something you cram in your face to get you to the next meal.

- Food stops being face entertainment.

- Food takes on a special place in your life to support your life as a foundation of physical health.

When you take the extra time to prepare your meals—and it will take extra time, and planning – you are preparing your medicine. The garlic oil recipe in this Liver Plan is the same garlic oil that you would put into your ear for an earache or paint on the Gargoyle bread recipe for a snack.

Garlic oil becomes your medicine when you put it in your ear and it becomes your Food as Medicine when you paint it on your bread. Same food, different job. That's the concept - Food as Medicine.

There are three types of food:

1) Don't touch it!

2) It's okay.

3) Food as Medicine

Here are a few food examples to further explain this concept:

Food as Medicine Example: Spaghetti sauce

1) Sauce with partially-hydrogenated oil or "spice" in the ingredient list is considered - - Don't touch it! POISON!

2) Sauce from the health food store with a few additives you can understand when you read the ingredient label, like tomatoes, onions, etc. is Okay food.

3) Homemade sauce from this book made with EVOO (extra virgin olive oil) and has homemade minced garlic is considered--Food as Medicine.

Salt Example:

Don't Touch it Salt:

1) <u>Iodized Salt</u> contains "sodium silicoaluminate which is a form of aluminum. This salt not only gives you iodide in the form of potassium iodide, but you are fed your daily allotment for aluminum. How much aluminum do you need every day. ZERO!

Aluminum is deadly! Don't cook with it. Don't cook in it. But, most importantly DON'T EAT iodized salt! The salt is bleached to make it stark white and the minerals have been stripped from it to sell to someone else for more profit. In a better language most will understand, this non-food product is similar to eating bleached white flour. Don't touch that either!

Table Salt: Morton Salt has salt without the word "Iodized" on it. This salt is bleached and the 90 trace minerals are stripped, too. Dangerous to man and beast! Don't touch it.

<u>Sea salt</u> – I bought sea salt from the Health Food Store and when I compared it to the table salt I had in the laundry room, (I use table salt to remove stains and it preserves colors on clothes.) it was as white as the table salt. The color of the salt seems to be a good way to know what you are buying. Bleached salt is not healthy.

Unfortunately, the label does not need to disclose if it was bleached. The FDA calls this additive "incidental additives." All salt in America is bleached and doesn't need to disclose this information. They assume we know? I'm the one with the Ph.D., and I didn't know. Integrity in the United States is bankrupt for a rich bank account.

Later, I bought Morton Natural Sea Salt. It was an off white color. That should be an indication that this salt is good. I called the one eight hundred number and the operator assured me that they do NOT bleach this salt.

It was twice as expensive as the Morton regular table salt, and the color was okay - so I thought it might be fine. I used this sea salt in my drinking water, and it gave me a big headache. (1/4 teaspoon per 32 ounces of water or one quart.) This is don't touch it salt, too.

Remember, I am the canary in a coal mine – that means I am very weak and/or very sensitive. My body shouts at me when I feed it something detrimental to my health. How does my body shout at me? I get a headache.

<u>Kosher Salt:</u> Don't touch it. The only difference is the coarseness of the salt, and it was blessed by a Rabbi. Sometimes this salt sometimes has yellow prussiate of soda added to it for freer flowing of the salt. This additive may produce a cyanide gas. Don't touch it!

2) I am sorry to report, but I cannot find okay salt for this Salt Example. Most salts are "don't touch it" food. If you are serious about getting well, get serious about your salt. Dr. Fereydoon Batmanghelidj, M.D. from his text called, "Your Body's Many Cries for Water" calls the salt most Americans eat as "a slow poison."

3) Celtic Sea Salt – Food as Medicine. This salt has a few ways to buy it. There is the light gray and the gray variety. You can also pick the coarseness of the salt with a fine ground or coarse salt.

In my opinion, this salt is Food as Medicine. I suggest it for adding the fine ground sea salt in your food recipes. No, this salt does NOT give me a headache. In fact, I notice that I have more energy and clearer thinking when I use it.

I use the coarse ground salt in Dr. B's Recipe. Let it sit for a minute and it is completely dissolved.

You can go to my website for more information and click the link so the Food as Medicine salt can be delivered to your home.

http://www.migrainephd.com/types-of-salt/

Food as Medicine Example: Corn:

1) Canned corn with sugar and/or any other ingredients - Don't touch it!

2) Frozen corn – Ingredients: corn – that's it. It's okay. It is only okay and will not heal you, but is okay for 20 percent of what you eat. Why? Because the plastic bag may leech into the corn and other veggies.

3) Fresh corn on the cob - Food as Medicine.

Are you getting a feel for this concept? What is my gauge? My gauge is the man-made processing. The more processing food goes through, the less food value it has. That is how food becomes "Don't touch it" - too much man-made processing.

The spices mentioned in this book are found in your local grocery store in the "Spice" section. When you have a choice, always buy the organic spices for having the best chance the spices are the best you can buy. You use a small amount and it is necessary to have the best.

Always read the ingredients on these, too. Food Manufacturers like to make special spice combinations that will taste better than what you have at home. Why do they taste better? Because Food Manufacturers use chemicals to make their products taste better. Simple and cheap chemicals for them, but deadly and expensive health care costs for you.

If your spice mentions any other ingredient than the ones asked for in this book, it is probably from the "Don't touch it" type of food. Be careful. Your health may be at risk. The "Food as Medicine" type of food should be eaten 80 percent of the time. 20 percent of the okay food. The Don't Touch it food should NEVER be eaten.

Stress:

Everyone is stressed about stress. What could be more stressful than when our nation was at war? In World War II, the enemy was parked off American shores! However, through all this stress, disease was at an all-time low. Why didn't stress from the War cause illness to increase during wartime?

Because the war efforts were priority, and food processing of white flour and white sugar were in short supply. In fact, sugar, coffee and fat were rationed. Result? Less disease. Disease and diet are related topics. The only people I know who are entirely stress free are all the people buried in the cemetery.

You must eat food for your medicine, and then you will not need less or no over-the-counter or prescription medicine because food will be your medicine. When Food is your Medicine, life's stresses does not hurt your health. Your body can handle most stress because your food will strengthen your health.

<u>Six Ways to Add EVOO to your diet:</u>

1) Toss hot or cold vegetables with two Tablespoons EVOO, a little garlic and/or fresh lemon juice. EVOO Salad Dressing tastes great over veggies!

2) Stir fry vegetables with two Tablespoons EVOO, two minced garlic cloves and a sprinkling of fresh herbs. (Never use the package of ingredients that comes with stir fry!! Lots and lots of chemicals in them.)

3) Rub potatoes with EVOO before baking for added crispness. I do NOT recommend eating the skin from a non-organic potato.

4) Add a Tablespoon of EVOO to filtered water without fluoride when boiling whole wheat pasta to prevent pasta from sticking to the pot. Toss cooked pasta with a Tablespoon or two of EVOO immediately after draining.

5) When broiling or roasting meats or poultry, brush EVOO to seal in natural juices.

6) Sauté homemade breadcrumbs with EVOO or Garlic EVOO and paprika. Cook until golden brown. Add on top of steamed vegetables and salads as a crunchy garnish.

My Discovery

When I was 27, my clothes were fitting tight. I didn't have the energy I had at 20. Friends and relatives told me - "Diana, get a grip. You have two small children, you are pushing 30. Relax and act your age."

"No way!" I shouted back to them. I began my health nut career by going to the library to get some facts. Sorry, no internet in the dark ages when I was 27. What did I learn? I had to get moving. Knowing I would NEVER go to an aerobic class at a gym unless I HAD to go, I decided to teach. I went to the best training, AFAA. (American Fitness Association of America) I became certified and began to teach an aerobic class at my church three times a week.

Of course that worked - until 20 years later I found my clothes fitting tight again. Hey, I was exercising - what gives? By this time my health was plagued with sinus headaches, TMJ and just being tired and achy most of the day. My sinus pills stopped working. I found myself in bed three or four times a week from a bad headache.

When I went to the medical doctor, he diagnosed me with migraines, and gave me prescription pain medication. I never took one of those pills that he said would enlarge the blood vessels of my brain to "manage" my pain. I didn't want to manage it, I wanted it to be GONE! Good-bye.

Friends and family didn't help - they kept saying, "Relax you are pushing 50. Act your age! This is normal?" YIKES, I didn't want to be "normal." I went back to doing some research and found Clayton College of Natural Health. I enrolled.

What I learned shocked me. Americans eat over nine pounds of food additives and preservatives in their food every year! That was enough for me. I went through my kitchen cabinets and cleared them out.

My guidelines for cleaning out my cabinets: Just one guideline: If I didn't understand the words in the ingredient list? Gone. I put the food into a box to be given to a homeless shelter that thought this food was good to eat.

My family thought I had lost my mind. When in reality, I had found my mind and was reclaiming my life. I deleted all the chemicals in my diet, and it immediately deleted 90 percent of my headaches. And now for a secret discovery besides ridding myself of illness. I lost 10 pounds without doing anything different. Yup, no exercise

Real Life Story:

Gloria:

"I threw up ten times; I thought I was going to die. Then I spoke to Dr. Rossano, and she told me that it was the food that I was eating."

Gloria started eating from the concepts in this book and in 48 hours, Gloria said,

"I'm a new woman since eating the way Dr. Rossano told me to eat."

What makes the Liver Cleanse Diet so special? The concept is so simple that it almost escaped me for several years. While I was studying for my Ph.D., the two-second answer to a healthier liver came to me.

> Man's processed food causes disease.
> God's whole, fresh food causes healing.

That's it. Simple, huh? Too simple.

Even my trusted Campbell's soup had a long, long list of words I couldn't understand. Maybe I should call my lawyer so he could explain? Instead, I called the Campbell's Soup's 1-800 telephone number.

The operator said,

> *"Our customers like the taste better*
>
> *when we add MSG to our products."*

Later, I read a report that Campbell's was one of the few Food Manufacturers that tried fewer chemicals in their foods, but profits went down. Here is the problem: "Customers like the taste better" is a true statement. Nevertheless, customers are not told that these same chemicals are making their immune system weak or confused, or like me--causing migraines and fibromyalgia. Your liver is in danger from this deadly additive that has over 13 different names - MSG.

In my opinion, there isn't anything on super market shelves that is more lethal than canned broth. It has so many chemicals in it, I dare say it is, without a doubt, NOT food. Canned broth is a chemical cocktail.

Do you think that if you use the recipe for chicken broth in this book that it will maintain your recipes to still taste fantastic? No, this won't work as a substitute with recipes that call for canned broth, because those recipes are relying on the "chemicals" to excite your brain into <u>thinking</u>, "Wow, this food tastes fantastic!"

So, if you want to be healthy, don't eat that Poison. The recipes in this book use other food to make your recipes taste good. Like what? Garlic, onions, slow cooking, cutting ingredients tiny and other basic cooking techniques.

Dr. Blaylock, a neuro-surgeon, believes that these chemicals are sometimes stored in the brain and promote brain tumors. (MSG was one of the main "triggers" that caused my migraines. MSG is deadly to your liver.)

Your immune system is on a constant search for invaders - that's its job. The question may arise: "Is that a chemical or a germ?" Hmmm, your body doesn't know. In order to be on the safe side, your body's immune system attacks "it" just in case.

Now, the health problems begin. You see the "it" wasn't a germ, but a part of your body. This could be the beginning of an autoimmune disease or other health problems.

My new diet discovery turned my whole world upside down! I was forced to re-think my entire eating and entertainment lifestyle. That was NOT easy. I loved eating out! I loved inviting our kids to meet us at our favorite restaurants. We would eat, visit, and then leave the mess for the restaurant staff to clean. We all had F-U-N, fun!

When I ate at home, I loved using the convenience foods. The bag of yellow rice and spices mixed together was easy and no fuss. The yellow rice was delicious every time, too. I loved the instant spaghetti sauce in a glass jar!

Making a food change was difficult. My pantry was full of foods that had chemicals in them. However, I could see a definite connection between the food I ate and my chronic pain. At first, I couldn't believe my discovery, but every time I went out to eat at a restaurant, my health would suffer and give me more proof that restaurant food and other processed foods were bad for my health.

What happened to me? I was awakened at three a.m. with a horrible migraine and then spent the entire next day suffering in bed. I hated that! Eating at a restaurant was fun, but nothing – I mean NOTHING was worth an entire day of pain.

For you, it may be different? Is your life worth more than just eating out? Can't you have the same amount of fun eating at home? Today, I have more fun eating at home because I know there won't be a surprise wake up call at three a.m. of pain. I found out that health is earned and NOT found in a pill, surgery or treatment.

Health is robbed by eating convenience foods combined with a fast, easy lifestyle. I saved time in the kitchen by eating out, but it was stolen from me when I was sick in bed for days from eating the processed man-made foods.

Bad Fats & Oils, Enemy #1

"Lettuce" (Let us) talk about the problems, Gimmicks. I do not like gimmicks. The Food Manufacturers are not naïve to the world of gimmicks. Like product labels on our grocery store shelves that boast- - "<u>NO FAT.</u>" The front of the label is called the "adver-teasing." It is "teasing" you that "NO FAT" is healthy by twisting the truth, just a little.

Many consumers are in a tizzy to lower their fat because of Healthy Hearsay. People quickly scoop the "No Fat" product up off the shelves without reading its ingredients. Now, here is the gimmick! The products that boast "no fat" usually contain partially hydrogenated oils that will raise your cholesterol levels! Nah! Can't be? Am I nuts? Advertisers fail to mention that little ditty! Nevertheless, it is a fact!

> "The strongest correlation for breast cancer has been with the intake of the trans fatty acids that are created when vegetable oils are hydrogenated to make margarine
>
> and solid vegetable shortening."
>
> Elson Haas, M.D.

Trans fatty acid is another word for partially hydrogenated oil. You will hear "trans fatty acid" mentioned in the news, BUT newscasters rarely call it hydrogenated oil. It is as if they do not want consumers to make the connection between trans fats and partially hydrogenated oil. Are we consumers mushrooms? Kept in the dark and fed horse manure? You bet. They want profits.

Dr. Walter Willett, Chairman of Nutrition at Harvard Medical, has published a paper on a 14-year study involving 85,000 nurses. It clearly shows that people consuming the most trans-fatty acids have the highest rate of heart disease.

Other researchers such as Dr. Henry Blackburn, professor at the University of Minnesota, and Dr. William Castelli, Director of the Framingham Cardiovascular Institute, have found the same findings. (More later on Dr. Castelli's findings on "Poison - Animal Products) There is also a link with trans-fatty acids (margarine, soybean oil, Crisco etc.) and diabetes:

> "By consuming "abnormally changed molecular essential fatty acids," abnormal proteins are produced by the body. The abnormal proteins cannot properly synthesize the insulin in its metabolic state. The insulin eventually becomes ineffective in reducing sugar in the blood stream."
>
> David Lawrence Dewey, a medical columnist

Those are scary statements. Why? Because partially hydrogenated and hydrogenated oils are in too many products to list! I went to the grocery store with my digital camera and photographed one hundred and fifty food products in just over an hour. Partially hydrogenated oil is in 90 percent of all processed food!

According to the Center for Science in Public Interest who analyzed 41 supermarkets and restaurant foods purchased in seven cities across the country, they found that restaurants have joined the ranks of using partially hydrogenated oil to prepare their food.

The Center for Science in Public Interest restaurant findings:

1) All the major restaurant chains use trans-fatty oils for their French fries. Burger King and Wendy's are the worst!

2) Red Lobster's Admiral's Feast dinner contains a two-day supply of artery-clogging oil.

3) KFC, formerly Kentucky Fried Chicken, (they changed their name) has only a day's supply of trans-fatty acid. Oooo, but still poison.

4) A Dunkin Donuts old-fashioned cake donut contains more bad fat than eight strips of bacon!

5) Campbell's soups are loaded with hydrogenated oils.

6) 99 percent of all store-bought cookies, crackers, chips, and pretzels all contain hydrogenated oil!

You cannot get away from partially hydrogenated oil! Changing this one dietary lifestyle could reduce heart disease by 43 percent, according to the Harvard School of Public Health. Deleting this one additive to your diet can add years to your life and years to the health of your liver.

Many countries have already banned this oil from their grocery store shelves. In fact, Denmark banned hydrogenated oils in the 1970's. It is interesting that Denmark has the lowest diagnosed rates of heart disease, cancers, diabetes, and autoimmune diseases than any other country in the world.

Russel Jaffe, M.D., a noted medical researcher stumbled across the fact that hog farmers wouldn't feed trans-fatty acids (hydrogenated oil) to their hogs. The reason? The hogs died when they ate it! That'll ruin your hog business! <u>FAST</u>!

When Dr. Jaffe contacted the U.S. Department of Agriculture concerning the death of hogs, they admitted they had known about it. However, it was not in their jurisdiction.

When Dr. Jaffe contacted the Food & Drug Administration, they simply said they didn't have time to investigate it. Every day our children eat store-bought crackers, cookies, and bread with this poison, man-made oil in it. The FDA doesn't have time to protect our children?

Okay, calm down. I was quite upset when I learned this information. Remember one thing, Food Manufacturers--are <u>NOT</u> out to get us. This is simply a money thing. Any business that wants to stay in business is always looking for ways to cut back on their overhead expenses and maximize profits. Hydrogenated oil is another way for Food Manufacturers to use cheap oil instead of expensive oils.

In addition to being cheap, hydrogenation extends shelf life. Perfect--for them, but not perfect for consumers. So, how do we eliminate hydrogenated oil from our grocery store shelves?

One of my seminar participants stood up and yelled with a clenched fist, "**<u>BOYCOTT</u>**! Let's make signs and walk up and down in front of grocery stores!" While I appreciated his understanding about the danger of eating this poison, I said, Nah! Here's a better way. You can vote. Didn't see it written on your voting ballot last November?

Nope, you have not seen it on your ballot, and there is an excellent chance that you will never see it on your voting ballot. So, what did I mean by vote?

Use your food budget to vote. No, we are not giving our food money away to politicians. Take your new knowledge to the grocery store. Now that you know that hydrogenated oils are unhealthy, do not buy them! That's it!

The next time you go to the grocery store, read the food labels of the products you usually purchase. The voting comes when you <u>DO NOT</u> buy any products with hydrogenated or partially hydrogenated oils in them. Your food dollars are your one and <u>only</u> vote!

If Americans got serious and wanted to eliminate hydrogenated oil from our grocery store shelves, they could do it. What is the biggest impact an individual can make on Food Manufacturers?

Decreased sales!

That is how consumers can hit Food Manufacturers right where it hurts. Reduce what is on their bottom line!

Health Problems Related to Hydrogenated Oil:

Migraine & other headaches

Diabetes
Heart Disease
Raised Cholesterol
Muscle spasms (Like TMJ, or lower back problems)
Liver problems

(Signs of an upset liver.)
Eczema (bad complexion, acne or pimples)
Foggy Thinking
No energy
Excessive weight gain or easy weight gain
Moody or depressed
Dry, red or itching eyes
Poor digestion
Nausea

Physical Warnings Brilliant red ear lobes.
Bright red cheeks.
Dark circles or puffy under the eyes.
Allergic eye wrinkles.
Nose is always stuffy or dripping.
Personality change. (Aggression or depression.)
Abdominal pain or bloating.

NOTE: It has been typical for most people who have eaten the Liver Cleanse Plan to lose weight. One seminar participant reported losing ten pounds just by eliminating hydrogenated oil from her diet. Why? Because the toxins are being released by their body's fat cells. Even athletic Christine, who is a personal trainer at the YMCA near my home, lost three pounds just by eliminating one toxin in her food - hydrogenated oil.

"I can't believe it, but I lost three pounds just by eliminating hydrogenated oil from my diet." Christine

Eating hydrogenated oil will contribute to higher cholesterol levels. Seventy-five percent of the cholesterol in our body is self produced. That is amazing! Have you ever wondered why your body makes so much cholesterol? Medical science tells us that without cholesterol, your body could not make your hormones. So, why are you bombarded with the entire scare about having too much cholesterol in your body?

Was God wrong when He made our bodies to make 75 percent of our body's total cholesterol? Are you ready for another theory? I can hear you say, "What do you mean another "theory?" Americans take cholesterol-lowering drugs based on mainstream health's theory. (pharmaceutical sales promote this theory)

If it were factual and not a theory, why would cholesterol test results change from year to year? One year a safe cholesterol reading is 220, and then later it changes to 200. That's an indication of a theory.

American medical schools teach our student doctors that a diet high in cholesterol is generally acknowledged to be the major component of arterial plaque, and plaque is related to heart disease. (This is the plaque theory. Yes, it is a theory, too. There is another heart disease theory in the "Poison --Animal Product" section that says heart disease is caused by a hormonal imbalance.)

Why the cholesterol theory does NOT make sense.

How do you make a dress? Yes, I know I changed the subject, but work with me here. Answer: With cloth, zipper, buttons, etc. Right? You do not buy a dress to make a dress, do ya? Nope.

Something for the guys, if you want to make a Ford, you do not buy a Ford. You buy a chassis, an engine, tires, seats, etc. Right? Right.

Okay, it is the same concept with our bodies. Our bodies do not make cholesterol from cholesterol. Our bodies make cholesterol from pancakes, syrup, and other foods. Therefore, eating foods that contain cholesterol is NOT the problem.

Here is the problem. Stop concentrating on reducing cholesterol levels in foods that contain cholesterol, and concentrate on reducing additives and preservatives in your food. Too much cholesterol is a sign that you are eating too many toxins. Like what? All the "Poison" on ingredient labels. Yes, hydrogenated oil is a toxin that raises cholesterol levels.

"In appearance, cholesterol is a soapy, yellowish-white type of fat that is an essential body-building block. It is the envelope that surrounds our body cells. The body can manufacture cholesterol with ease, but about 25 percent of the cholesterol in the body comes from the food we eat."

Francisco Contreras, M.D., believes that God had it all together when He made our bodies to manufacture its own cholesterol.

> "Cholesterol is a trapper of toxins. It surrounds toxins."
>
> Francisco Contreras, M.D.

That means that cholesterol may be considered as part of our immune system. The immune system's job is to protect our bodies from germs and to gobble them up for removal. Our white blood cells are responsible for this "clean up" job. If a person is eating too many additives and preservatives, then their body will produce more cholesterol to "surround toxins" for their removal. Makes sense?

If you want to decrease cholesterol, try eating foods as God designed especially for His children. What are God's foods? God's foods are fresh fruits and vegetables, whole grains, nuts, seeds and legumes (that's beans). Cholesterol is a good thing:

> "Most people have a negative impression of cholesterol, but it is actually one of the most vital substances in your body, essential for building of your cell walls and your nerve sheaths."
>
> Mitchell L. Gaynor, M.D.

> "Cholesterol is made in the liver, skin, adrenal glands, intestines, aorta, and testicles. Cholesterol is so vital to your survival that if you don't consume any cholesterol in your diet, your dozen little cholesterol factories cook it up out of fat, protein, or carbohydrate. So, reducing your cholesterol level is a hopeless struggle."
>
> David Reuben, M.D.

Dr. Francisco Contreras' theory is that the body makes an abundance of cholesterol to fight an abundance of toxins in the body. The more toxins, the more cholesterol the body manufactures. With this new theory in mind, a body creating too much cholesterol means trouble.

Your liver is being poisoned by hydrogenated or partially hydrogenated oil. Both of these oils are responsible for poisoning your liver!

Yes, your doctor is correct, too much cholesterol is a health warning. On the other side of the coin, too little cholesterol is a health warning that may be linked to getting cancer.

"Research has been fairly consistent showing a relationship of low blood cholesterol value and cancer."

Edward R. Pinckney, M.D.

This new theory gives God credit for making our body correctly.

* Too little cholesterol is a liver that is in trouble and unable to keep up making cholesterol to fight disease. This is a sign of an immune system NOT working. If your immune system stops working, you are setting yourself up for getting cancer. Your liver is the key player for avoiding cancer.

* Too much cholesterol is sign of a liver that is in trouble and making cholesterol to remove the toxins from the body.

So, my question is, "Why is your body making too much cholesterol?" Is the answer for high cholesterol a prescription drug that will put more toxins into the body? All prescription medication AND over the counter medicine is liver toxic.

Edward R. Pinckney, M.D. calls cholesterol drugs,

"Dangerous, and totally useless."

According to Max Gerson, M.D., cancer develops because the body's liver is clogged and cannot purify the blood. Low cholesterol levels would be linked to cancer because the liver is not able to do its job.

What's one of the four hundred jobs the liver has to do? Make cholesterol to fight toxins. Again, this points to the fact that God made us correctly when He gave our bodies the ability to make cholesterol. Cholesterol fights toxins for removal out of the body.

Toxins come in many forms. Fumes are toxins when pumping gas into your car. Toxins could be chemicals you handle at work and may be absorbed through your skin. Be careful when you spray roach spray in the house because you can absorb the poisons from the spray through your skin and lungs.

LaSalle D. Leffall, M.D., Howard University College of Medicine, says:

* one-to-two percent of cancer is from air pollution (like pumping gas in your car)

* four-to-five percent is from the work place environment (like breathing hair spray in a beauty salon)

* sixty-six percent of all cancer is from cigarette smoking and what you eat (like additive-filled, and processed foods.)

You have control of smoking and what you eat. Dr. Leffall is telling us that cancer is caused by lifestyle, not heredity. If you have high cholesterol, you need to find out why your body is producing too much toxin-fighting cholesterol.

Chemical additives in your food may be triggering your body to make too much cholesterol. You must eliminate those toxins. If you think eggs are toxic because they have high cholesterol, think again.

My student, Peggy came to see me because she wanted to have more energy. She loved eggs, and when I told her that eating four or five free-range chicken eggs a week was fine - she did. She stopped eating chemicals in her diet and loved eating a more whole food diet. After a month, her husband panicked and suggested that Peggy have her cholesterol checked.

Peggy said, "My cholesterol has been 220 for about three years. This time it was 152. Since my good report, my husband is open to eating this way, too."

What toxins are you consuming? If you are eating out, you are at the mercy of restaurant owners--people running a business. Don't forget their first concern is for high profits, not for healthy customers. They have payroll to meet. Store rent to pay and all the other hefty expenses for running a business.

Restaurant owners want fast and cheap food to sell at a maximum profit. Ingredients? Nah, customers don't ask what's in the food, so why bother putting in expensive ingredients! Use chemicals to make cheap food taste great. Use lots and lots of prepared foods to save preparation time in their kitchen, (this saves on payroll) and nobody complains.

Owners smile all the way to the bank. Customers groan all the way to the doctor's office. Then, it's the doctor's time to smile all the way to the bank.

Read your food contract!! Remember, the front of the label is the "adver-teasing." If you want to read your contract, read the "ingredient list." Switch to extra virgin olive oil. EVOO will lower your cholesterol. EVOO is good fat. Don't eat any other oil, because of the man-made processing it is bad fat.

It is too difficult to investigate each oil and call each oil manufacturer to find out how the oil was made. Besides, I have tried calling Food Manufacturers - it doesn't work. The operator has a script to read and the script doesn't make any sense to me.

EVOO, or extra virgin olive oil, is just that--"virgin," untouched, and unprocessed by man. It's one of the only oils that are still manufactured "purely." If it doesn't say "virgin," don't eat it. "Extra Light Olive Oil" is more twisting of words by Food Manufacturers. Don't eat it. This is a bad fat.

If you must eat butter - preferably eat non-hormone butter, but use it sparingly. Read the ingredient list on the butter. Yes, there is one. You prefer "ingredients: Pasteurized Organic Sweet Cream (milk) Microbial culture."That's it. No flavoring and no salt. By the way, none of my recipes use butter. Yup, none.

Are you still confused by food labels? Go to my website: http://www.migrainephd.com/read-food-labels/

When buying butter, check the ingredient's label. Natural flavoring is a common man-made additive to butter. Natural flavoring could be MSG. When you eat butter make sure it says, "Organic." I never eat butter. EVOO is a great HEALTHY substitute to eating butter.

How to Lower Your Cholesterol Test Numbers:

*Adapted from Cathey Pinckney and Edward R. Pinckney, M.D., Do-it-yourself Medical Testing.

1) Have blood taken from your vein. (Finger-stuck blood gives a higher reading.)

2) Sit in a chair. (Standing could easily make results 50 points higher than sitting.)

3) Make sure the chair is comfortable and you are as relaxed as possible when you are having this test done. (You may get a higher cholesterol test result if you rush to the test or are emotionally upset before the test.)

4) Try not to take any prescription or over-the-counter drugs before your test. Aspirin, for example, is one drug that can change cholesterol values.

NOTE: Ask your doctor if any of the prescription drugs you take will change cholesterol test values before discontinuing the drug.

5) Taking female hormones will lower blood cholesterol values.

6) Twenty-four-hours before your test, be especially aware of your diet. A controlled fast of fresh fruits and vegetables will balance your body in preparation for the test.

7) Stop eating chemicals in your food and switch to EVOO.

Sugar, Liver Enemy #2

The most popular additive in the United States is refined, white sugar. Is it food? No, refined, white sugar is not food - it's an additive or "liver enemy." The sugar cane plant is food, and workers who pick it, chew on it while they work do not suffer health problems from this plant. In its whole food state, raw sugar cane plant is food. (Don't be confused with a product called,

> *"Sugar in the Raw." Sugar in the raw is 95% refined as regular white sugar. (George Wootan, M.D.)*

"It takes a quart and a half of cane juice to make a single teaspoon of refined sugar," George Wootan, M.D., Take Charge of Your Child's Health.

That's a lot of reducing to make the healthy cane juice into deadly sugar! After this intense processing, sugar has no essential nutrients left in it. When you eat refined sugar, your body robs stored vitamins and minerals from itself in order to balance the unbalanced refined sugar you just ate.

Fructose is more refined than white sugar. No, it's not natural. It sounds healthy and Food Manufacturers put fructose in most cranberry and other fruit juices or fruit drinks. Fructose makes you fat faster than table sugar. Both sugar and fructose will cause your body to become unbalanced and will lead to illness or loss of energy. Too much of this refined sugar may be a trigger for migraine headaches, liver problems, autoimmune problems, high blood pressure, tooth decay, and emotional or obsessive eating disorders.

In 1821, each person in America ate an average of 10 pounds of refined, white sugar a year. In 1993, that amount increased to 147 pounds of white sugar and 50 pounds of fake, man-made sugar a year. That's a total of 197 pounds per person! No wonder 61 percent of adults are obese in the United States.

Sugar consumption increases every year in America. The outcome of our overindulgence is much more than just empty calories with overweight adults and children. It seems that illness increases along with sugar consumption increase.

The Nutrition Action Newsletter writes:

"We are drowning in liquid candy."

Soft drinks are contributing to many health problems in America. Did you know that a diet high in sugar can contribute to depression? Here are some interesting facts about kids and depression:

NOTE: Clinical depression is the most common mental health problem in the U.S. Please don't be confused with depression as a day or two feeling "blue" or "under the weather." Clinical depression lasts a minimum of two weeks.

"Seven-to-fourteen percent of children will experience an episode of clinical depression before the age of 15!"

YIKES! Children six-to-twelve years old used 51,000 prescriptions for Prozac in 1995, and in 1996, that number increased by 209%! (This doesn't take into account other name-brand and generic medications prescribed for depression - just Prozac.)

"Sugar causes a child's immune system to go into slow motion,"
Robert Mendelsohn, M.D.

Professor Low, a biochemist who suffered from migraine headaches for over thirty years, undertook his own research project. He uncovered ample evidence that migraine is a biochemical disorder that can be treated and controlled by diet. (Just like me and Max Gerson, M.D.)

Professor's Low's research of twenty years pointed to refined sugar being the biggest enemy to the migraine sufferer. He discovered that the blood sugar levels were directly responsible for his migraines.

"(Sugar) is a drug because I think it is easily the most commonly addictive food/drug worldwide."
Elson Haas, M.D.

With this in mind, if you have diabetes or hypoglycemia, your disease could be directly connected to how much refined foods you eat. You must stop eating all fake and refined sugars. Don't eat enriched food products. Yes, that means zero. Refined or fake sugar is NOT healthy for anyone.

Keeping your food balanced will keep the health of your liver balanced. The more you eat balanced, unrefined food, the less your body will crave refined, processed foods. I used to love banana splits. After eating the Liver Cleanse Plan for about six months, I could eat about five or six bites of a banana split before I was "sugared out" and had to put my spoon down.

Today, I can say "no" easily because I don't "want" sugar anymore. This has nothing to do with my strong self control!

Mary Ellen and her husband, Phil, would have ice cream as their evening snack ritual. Since they have been eating whole foods on the Liver Cleanse Plan, they have a raw apple or fruit salad as their evening treat.

"I'm very surprised, but we don't miss our evening ice cream. I didn't read this book to lose weight, but I've lost 13 pounds in about four weeks." Mary Ellen (After three months, Mary Ellen's fibromyalgia was in total remission, and she lost 25 pounds.)

"I would die for Krsipy Kreme donuts; they are my favorites. But, now I realized - you will die for them. Since I've been eating this way, food odors at the mall don't tempt me anymore. I've lost 15 pounds in about four weeks." Phil
NOTE:

Phil is diabetic and his fasting blood sugar went from 200 to 130 in about two weeks. Throw away your refined sugar in the sugar bowl. I have Celtic sea salt in my sugar bowl. Raw honey is a better sweetener or grade A maple syrup. Sugar is a liver enemy and will destroy your liver.

Enriched Foods, Liver, Enemy #3

Enriched Flour makes Our Daily Bread into Our Daily Poison: Have you noticed that kids seem to need braces earlier and earlier? Maybe you got braces at 16 years old, but your children may them earlier? A contributing factor is enriched bread and other enriched food products in the American diet.

Our bread has 23 essential nutrients robbed from it. Then the bread has chemicals added to ensure its long shelf life. Consequently, our daily bread has become our daily poison. Bread in America is unbalanced and therefore not food.

They sell the bran part of the flour for horse feed, and the hull part goes for pig feed. Americans eat the garbage part of the wheat. We are the richest nation on the planet and we eat the garbage of the planet.

In other places around the world, people buy their bread daily because they do not want chemicals or preservatives in their bread like Americans eat.

Enriching our bread takes out all of the chromium. Without chromium, your body cannot successfully balance or maintain its blood-sugar level. Put another way, white, enriched food products make you fat because it lacks chromium for you to digest the enriched food. Your body continues to rob itself of chromium, until you become fat. Enriched foods make you fat because it is unbalanced food. This lack of chromium contributes to getting diabetes.

Reading a bread label requires a degree as a food chemist. Consumers think that wheat flour is the same as whole-wheat flour. Not so. Most whole-wheat flour is only 10% whole wheat.

Enriched wheat flour is really bleached white flour with a few chemical nutrients put back to replace the many nutrients that have been processed out of the wheat. If it doesn't say <u>100%</u> whole wheat on the ingredient list, it's enriched. Then Food Manufacturers add dough conditioners, food colorings, and hydrogenated oil in our bread and call it "Health Nut." The only nut is you and I for trusting Food Manufacturers while they make a profit from what we buy at the grocery store.

Professor Roger Williams and his colleagues at the University of Texas did important experiments with "enriched" bread. They fed 64 laboratory rats "enriched" bread from weaning on. After three months, two thirds of the rats were dead. Yes, I said, dead. One third of the rats that survived all had growth abnormalities-tumors.

If enriched bread cannot keep a rat - an adaptive animal healthy, how can enriched bread grow a healthy child with strong bones and straight teeth? Henry A. Schroeder, M.D. in the U.S, and by M.O. Bruker in Germany, M.D. have listed 22 of the ingredients removed from all enriched bread:

<u>11 minerals are lost in refining flour:</u>
<u>Calcium 60%</u>
<u>Chromium 40%</u>
<u>Cobalt 89%</u>
<u>Copper 68%</u>

Iron 76%
Magnesium 85%
Molybdenum 48%
Phosphorous 71%
Potassium 77%
Selenium 16%

11 other nutrients lost in refining flour:
Strontium 95%
Zinc 78%
Vitamins B3, B2 and B3 72-81%
Vitamin B6 72%
Pantothenic acid 50%
Folacin 67%
Vitamin E 86%
Linoleic acid 95%
Protein 33%
Fiber 95%

If the dentist wanted to remove 22 of your teeth and give you back seven little false teeth, what would you do? You would spring right out of that chair and RUN out of the office — right? Would you call your mouth "enriched?" Of course not.

In 1936, an Ohio dentist, Weston Price, took an around-the-world trip of 150,000 miles. He thought that food grown in higher altitudes caused it to be more nutritious and wanted to prove his theory. What he found out was mind boggling. Dr. Price's research found that the food's altitude had nothing to do with how nutritious the food was for the people.

In 14 cultures, their diets ranged from the Swiss with exceptionally high vitamin dairy products, with meat once a week and vegetables, to Eskimo tribes wandering to follow the moose and caribou herds for their only source of food - meat. All who ate from the land were almost immune to dental problems.

In 14 cultures out of 14, there was one diet change that caused dental arch deformity and cavities to become epidemic among the natives. What was it? When the people deviated from their natural food and eating from the good of their land and ate "modern" man-made processed foods.

In 1936 Dr. Price said,

"The most universal disease in the world is the decay of the teeth. I have found that when the primitive people eat as we do, their teeth decay as ours do. I come to you as a missionary from them that you might learn of their accumulated wisdom because we're adding too much white flour and white sugar to our food. You, too, can have strong healthy bodies if you eat as they do."

Here is a link to hear Dr. Price for yourself.

http://www.migrainephd.com/is-sugar-poison/

The Price-Pottenger Association has the complete video story of Dr. Price's work available. 1-800-366-3748.

When anyone tells you how much protein or how many carbs (carbohydrates) you should eat – smile – then RUN! According to Dr. Weston Price's research, that information means nothing—zero.

Bottom line from Dr. Price's research?

Don't eat modern foods: enriched crackers, breads, pasta, or baked goods from 99% of restaurants and grocery stores. It is not food. The Liver Cleanse Plan has no white flour and no white sugar. Eat God's whole, unprocessed foods for a "strong, healthy body."

God's Whole Foods = Health
Man-made Processed Foods = Illness

Chemicals, Enemy #4

Generally Recognized as Safe (GRAS) The GRAS list was established in 1958 by Congress. In my opinion, this list is a waste of time to read because all food chemicals are dangerous chemicals- even salt because it is bleached. God never designed His children to eat anything but HIS food - as any designer would do. Do your best to eliminate chemicals what you ingest to as close to zero as possible.

Chemicals in your food contribute to the ill health of your liver because your liver must filter everything that enters your mouth out of the blood. Many chemicals have been approved for use in cosmetic products but these same approvals apply to Food Manufacturers and what they are allowed to put into our food. The FDA guidelines see no difference between IN your body or ON your body. Scary.

A few GRAS (generally accepted as safe) chemicals are benzoic acid, sodium benzoate, and BHA. David Reuben, M.D., names these as prime culprits to high blood pressure. Benzoic acid also has another warning attached to it from Aubrey Milunsky, M.D.:

> "In pregnant rats, the frequency of birth defects can be increased if aspirin is given together with benzoic acid."
> Aubrey Milunsky, M.D., Choices not Chances

If you are pregnant or planning to become pregnant, be careful eating any chemicals in your food. Benzoic acid is a common preservative in processed foods, but not common in God's creation (your body.) In other words, - you are eating a liver poison.

Americans eat chemicals in their food every day. There are new chemical foods being fabricated all the time. Food Manufacturers are motivated by the sound of the cash register – music to their ears. Because these chemicals are ingested - taken right into the body - they are the worst toxins in our world today! Processed foods are loaded with chemicals, preservatives, and flavor enhancers.

> *"Man-made food is the worst pollution and health hazard in America."*
> William Manahan, M.D.

Some of these "health hazards" are listed on the ingredient listing, and some are not. Chemicals, additives, artificial colors, and other undesirable "liver enemy" is put into our food that the FDA calls "standards of identity" and it is not required to be on the ingredient list because it has been "established" as "permissible ingredients" or "incidental additives" for a given product.

Autoimmune disease is nearly epidemic, and the cause may be linked to this food-additive pollution because the body cannot identify these foreign chemicals.

> *"Your body may learn to regard a particular food additive as an inappropriate and dangerous invader on your intestinal shore, and every time you eat that additive or preservative you may experience discomfort or loss of energy without necessarily knowing the cause."*
>
> Mitchell L. Gaynor, M.D.

"Liver enemy" - Unbalanced Caffeine

Approximately, 60 million Americans, two-thirds of whom are under 65, suffer from hypertension (high blood pressure) because of dehydration caused by unbalanced caffeine. Medication is given to relieve the symptoms of hypertension, but does little to address the cause. What is a contributing cause?

The main contributing cause of high blood pressure is a diet that is filled with drinking caffeine drinks, and NOT drinking enough filtered water without fluoride to obtain balance. High blood pressure is erased when the body receives enough water. What is enough water? Fifty percent of your body weight should be replenished by drinking water every single day.

If you drink caffeine and don't balance it with more water that is robbed by the caffeine, then you are poisoning your liver. An eight ounce caffeine drink will rob approximately twenty-four ounces of water from the body.

Our body is 75 percent water, and if an American drinks two glasses a day, they are exceptional water drinkers. Only problem - silent dehydration will contribute to high blood pressure, liver illness and obesity to name a few illnesses.

Ease Blood Pressure Tips:

- Drink more filtered water without fluoride every day. Fifty percent of your body weight.

- When you drink caffeine, drink more disilled water after the caffeine drink – approximately three times more water than caffeine drink or skip caffeine.

- Eat more fiber. (That means 100 percent whole grains, and don't eat enriched anything). Eat more beans, whole, fresh foods, nuts, and seeds.)

- Eat garlic. Garlic strengthens your immune system and lowers blood pressure.

- Eat EVOO (extra virgin olive oil) because we know the processing is "virgin" or "untouched by man."

- Stop drinking alcohol. Alcohol robs water from your body in the same way that caffeine robs the water. When you drink alcohol, drink more filtered water without fluoride after the alcohol drink – approximately three times more water than alcohol drink or skip it.

Decaffeinated coffee is a big "No-no." Why? Because Food Manufacturers use too many chemicals to remove the caffeine.

Coffee - should you indulge? Take this caffeine quiz and find out:

1) I need coffee to get started in the morning?

2) Do I need coffee as a pick me up?

3) Do I have health problems: high blood pressure, liver disease, kidney or bladder problems, or any health problem that causes me to see a doctor regularly or take medication?

If you answered "yes" to any one of these questions, indulging in one cup of coffee is "most likely NOT good for you." You should ask your doctor. He knows best.

If you don't have any health problems, one cup a day won't hurt, BUT—— don't get excited, there are some simple guidelines:

<u>One</u>: Don't drink decaf. I read that Food Manufacturers may use as many as 32 chemicals to release the caffeine from the coffee bean. The caffeine is natural to the coffee bean, leave it alone. Drink the "leaded" (with caffeine) version. If you have problems with digestion because of too little hydrochloric acid, a cup of coffee will encourage your stomach to make more hydrochloric acid (HCl.)

<u>Two</u>: Check the ingredient label. Puh-leeze—no natural flavor or flavoring. That could indicate that the Food Manufacturer is adding chemicals to your coffee. God's coffee bean in its natural unprocessed form is okay. Keep the ingredients: "100% coffee" and make sure the coffee beans have not been presoaked before you buy them. If the coffee is flavored or smells like a flavoring, that means the beans were presoaked. Avoid this coffee!

<u>Three</u>: Compensate for the diuretic effect of the caffeine and drink extra filtered water without fluoride to compensate. One

cup of coffee means you should drink four extra cups of filtered water without fluoride.

<u>Four</u>: Do not eat chemicals in your food. Be especially aware of benzoic acid, sodium benzoate, and BHA if you have high blood pressure.

<u>Five</u>: Stop smoking. (Smoking constricts blood vessels – more than coffee.) Some of my students reported to me that eating less chemicals in their food reduced their urge to smoke.

<u>Six</u>: Exercise: A 20-minute walk every day will improve your blood pressure and your mood.

"Liver enemy" – Chemicals MSG--Monosodium Glutamate

Chemicals have become commonplace in Americans' food. Here's a shocking statistic:

"The average American eats about

nine pounds of preservatives in their food every year."

Michael Colgan, Ph.D.

It is a challenge to find a salad dressing without MSG at your local grocery store. Many recipe books call for Dijon mustard, ketchup, Worcestershire sauce, or canned chicken broth. All of these prepared foods have MSG in them. Don't see it on the ingredient list? Look for artificial flavoring or natural flavorings.

Most brands have MSG in them. Deadly to your liver -don't eat it. Don't be fooled by words like, "Spice, Natural and Artificial Flavoring." All could be MSG.

Even your trusted tuna fish may have "vegetable broth" that could be another sneaky name for MSG. What is MSG? MSG, monosodium glutamate, is a drug that confuses your brain to make you "think" the food tastes great. MSG causes severe irreversible brain damage in baby mice, rats, chicks, and monkeys. Many medical doctors think MSG causes permanent brain damage in children, too.

Food Manufacturers want big bottom line profits and do not care if their foods cause your bottom to be big!

> *"MSG can cause severe irreversible brain damage in baby mice, rats, chicks, and monkeys."*
> David Reuben, M.D.

> *"The amount of MSG in a single bowl of commercially available soup is probably enough to cause blood glutamate levels to rise higher in a human child than levels that predictably cause brain damage in immature animals."*
>
> John Olney, M.D.

There's more MSG horror, but this information is kept far from the public's eye.

> *"(This) critical information is buried in technical and scientific journals, far from the public's eye."*
>
> Russell L. Blaylock, M.D.

Why "far from the public's eye?" Because these taste enhancers help cheap food taste scrumptious. Food Manufacturers buy cheap ingredients, add some chemicals, and the food tastes great. High profits. Long shelf life. Life is good.

In fact, there is a lobbying group called The Glutamate Association that has representatives from major U.S. Food Manufacturers such as Campbell and the Ajinomoto Company, which is the chief manufacturer of MSG and hydrolyzed vegetable protein. This is a billion-dollar business. Did you hear that? I didn't say a million-dollar business, I said **BILLION -DOLLAR BUSINESS**! These companies have plenty of money to keep the facts from us naive and trusting consumers!!

Here are some of the facts: God made our bodies like a chemistry set. A balance of chemicals in our brains helps us to think and bring about our feelings - happy and sad. When we eat man-made chemicals, they directly enter our body. Where do these chemicals go once we eat them?

Chemicals are foreign to our body, so our body has the task of doing <u>SOMETHING</u> with this <u>LIVER POISON!</u> Sometimes our body stores some of this POISON in our fat cells, and other times we don't know what the body will do. It is conceivable that these chemicals could interact and react with our own neurotransmitters in our brain.

Fat is NOT our enemy: the chemicals stored in the fat is our enemy.

"It is thought that the major portion of the "barrier" lies in the tight junction between the cells (endothelial cells) that line the capillary walls."

Russell L. Blaylock, M.D.

That's why the bulk of the chemicals we eat are stored in our fat storage and not in our brain. The blood-brain barrier (an invisible place in the body that protects the brain from chemical warfare. Each time a person eats MSG, this blood barrier becomes weaker and compromised and access to the brain becomes easier.

By compromised, I mean that the chemical MSG got past the gatekeeper (blood brain barrier) and entered the brain to stimulate the brain's pleasure area. Ahhhh, the food tastes great.

MSG is a drug that stimulates the brain.

When the blood-brain barrier is continually broken, lethal chemicals can enter our brain! Everyone knows that alcohol, a chemical, kills brain cells! Did you know that chemicals in our food kills brain cells, too? Not only do these chemicals kill brain cells, but here's a shocker!

"..from 1973 to 1990 brain tumors in people over the age of sixty-five have increased 67%."

Russell L. Blaylock, M.D.

Brain tumors could be your body's way of storing chemicals in your brain. A headache is always a warning sign from your body that something is wrong.

Please note for pregnant moms:

"In the developing baby, we know that not only does glutamate pass through the placental barrier into the baby's brain, but that drastic changes occur within the chemistry of the baby's

immature brain that effect not only the child's future behavioral development, but also its capacity to learn complex information. I warn all pregnant women to avoid all forms of glutamate and aspartame, especially aspartame."

Russell L. Blaylock, M.D.

"Liver enemy" – Chemicals -Aspartame

Aspartame or NutraSweet is found in Jell-O, toothpaste, breath mints and many unsuspecting candies and ice cream that boast being low in calories. Check the labels of everything before you put anything in your mouth!

TV dinners and other prepared foods are notorious for using man-made, fake sugar. Why? Because it is a cheaper ingredient.

"Most prepared TV dinners are known to lose up to 40 percent of their vitamin A, all of the vitamin C, 80 percent of all the B-complex vitamins, and over half of the vitamin E. You could almost get more nutrition by sucking on the wrapper."

David Rueben, M.D.

That's funny! "Suck on the wrapper." Wrappers on prepared foods that boast "low fat," "vitamin C added" or "low cholesterol" are "Healthy Hearsay" verbiage should make a loud bell go off in your head saying, "<u>DON'T EAT IT!</u>" or "<u>BEWARE!</u>"

"Liver enemy" – Chemicals - Aluminum

We know that one of the prevailing theories for the cause of Alzheimer's disease is chronic exposure to and its absorption of aluminum by the brain. But, did you know Alzheimer's Disease patients also have high levels of calcium and low levels of magnesium?

Dr. Blaylock believes that low levels of magnesium allow the blood-brain barrier to be susceptible to compromise. When the blood-brain barrier is broken, aluminum and other chemicals are allowed to enter the brain and do its damage. Magnesium is supposed to be in our Table salt, but it has been stripped away from the refining process and then bleached. Celtic Sea salt has magnesium in it because it is unrefined.

Killing brain cells (which accounts for neuro-degenerative diseases like Alzheimer's) and by storing the chemicals in the brain (which accounts for some brain tumors.)

Let's investigate a little more about autopsy results of Alzheimer's patients. What could cause the magnesium levels to be low? One reason for low magnesium might be eating calcium supplements. Americans do <u>NOT</u> have trouble eating calcium in their diets, but Americans <u>DO</u> have trouble absorbing that calcium. The media wants us to supplement calcium. Why? Because they sell calcium, that's why. Taking a calcium supplements may cause a magnesium imbalance.

What causes low levels of magnesium besides taking a calcium supplement? Prescription medications deplete magnesium levels in the body. Beta-blockers, high blood pressure medication and diuretics are just a few.

What might be another contributing cause for high aluminum levels? Cooking with aluminum cookware because the metal comes off into the food. Here's an experiment, try using a scouring pad on an aluminum pot. You will see some aluminum come off right before your eyes onto the pad. Scary, where is that residue going?

Many processed foods have been cooked in aluminum, and will be absorbed into your body when you eat the food. Most restaurant food is cooked in aluminum. Aluminum cookware is cheap, light weight and scours up to look very clean. Eating at all restaurants (not just fast-food restaurants) is like taking an aluminum supplement with your chemical food.

Canned and processed foods contain iodized salt. Iodized salt, some baking powders, alum in store-bought pickles are more known aluminum contaminants. Read food labels. Check your deodorant for aluminum because it may be absorbed through your skin.

"Thank you, Dr. Rossano, for opening my eyes. I was headed down the wrong path." Peggy.

"Liver enemy – Chemicals - Artificial, Natural, and Other Flavors

If your food label says, "natural flavor" added, is it food? Food is supposed to have flavor on its own - right? Food labels are sometimes vague because Food Manufacturers are not interested in educating you about their trade secrets. Artificial flavors, natural flavors, flavoring, or many other names could be MSG in your food!

"MSG and related toxins are added to foods in disguised forms. For example, among the Food Manufacturers favorite disguises are "hydrolyzed vegetable protein," "vegetable protein," "natural flavors," and "spices." Each of these may contain from 12% to 40% MSG."

George Schwartz M.D., "In <u>Bad Taste: The MSG Syndrome</u>"

"Extract" is another name for a set of chemicals being put into your food that sounds innocent. I found this out the hard way. How? Well, you see I am the proverbial canary. Don't understand?

Many years ago my grandfather worked in a coal mine, miners would bring a canary down into the mine with them to test the air. If the canary fell to the bottom in its cage, the miners would evacuate the mine because toxic gases were being released that killed the canary. Why?

The canary has a very small lung capacity. This would make the canary the first to react to the toxic air long before the miners' health would be affected. I am the canary for humans. When the food is foul, I fall to the bottom of the cage, (my bed) with a headache.

How did I find out that extract is just another name for chemicals? Well, I was experimenting with the "Create-a-Cookie" recipe and bought extracts to try different flavors for cookies. The next morning, I awoke with a horrible headache, and thought, "That's weird." The second time I finally realized what I had done.

I'm so optimistic! I thought "extract" meant boiling down the peppermint leaves to make a concentrated extract? Thus, this same "trusting" and "naive" philosophy was how I contracted migraine headaches in the first place! I was trusting Food Manufacturers to make my food healthy! I made a bad choice. You, too?

A few more innocent-sounding additives found listed in <u>Real Food, Fake Food and Everything In Between</u> by Geri Harrington.

1) cooked apple

2) lemon oil

3) coffee concentrate

4) oil nutmeg

5) cola emulsion

6) apple cinnamon

7) butter emulsion

8) apple essence

They sound trustworthy to me, but that's exactly what Food Manufacturers designed - innocent sounding and fictitious names to unsuspecting victims--I mean, consumers.

<u>Mayonnaise:</u>

Question: Mayonnaise stays in the fridge and always tastes great. It never goes bad—one month, one year, it doesn't matter! Why?

Answer: Because mayonnaise and other "taste-good" sauces are not food—they are sauce chemicals. Real food goes bad. I have shoes in my closet that will go bad in less time than the mayo, ketchup and mustard will go bad. I don't want to eat my shoes, but why do I eat those condiments? Something worth thinking about the next time you use a refrigerator door condiment.

Here is one of the worst ingredients in the Mayo, it has hydrogenated oil in it!

Throw Store-Bought Mayo in the trash!

Instead of mayonnaise try this:

- Lightly paint or dip one side of the bread with some EVOO (Extra Virgin Olive Oil)
- Paint or drizzle some EVOO salad dressing on the bread.
- Lightly sprinkle the bread with basil or oregano.

Condiments and Chemicals:

Monosodium Glutamate or MSG has alias names:

1) Hydrolyzed Vegetable Protein
2) Hydrolyzed Protein
3) Hydrolyzed Plant Protein
4) Plant Protein Extract
5) Sodium Caseinate

6) Calcium Caseinate

7) Yeast Extract

8) Textured Protein

9) Autolyzed Yeast

10) Hydrolyzed Oat flour

All these are MSG alias names. Just chemicals, no protein, no yeast, no oat flour just plain chemicals that kill brain cells. All very dangerous to your liver!

The Following Chemicals May Have MSG hidden in them:

Malt extract, Malt Flavoring, Bouillon, Broth Stock, Flavoring, Natural Flavoring, Artificial Flavoring, Natural Beef or Chicken Flavoring, Seasoning, Spices.

NOTE:

Food Manufacturers use two very innocent chemical names in their products called, "Natural Flavoring" and "Artificial Flavoring." Think about it, if your food needs flavor, is it food? Sounds like your food is dead and the Food Manufacturer is trying to revive it.

Another "vague" chemical is "Spice." What kind of spice? If a Food Manufacturer is vague, it's because they don't want you to know their secrets. Their secrets are dangerous to your health. Most condiments have "spice" in them, but there's a very good chance the spice is MSG. Read food ingredient labels or better yet? Don't eat foods that have labels.

In George R. Schwartz, M.D.'s 1988 book, "In Bad Taste, The MSG Syndrome," he offers a list of "Monosodium Glutamate Aliases:

Accent, Ajinomoto, Zest, Vetsin, Gourmet powder, Subu, Chinese Seasoning, Glutavene, Glytacyl, RL-50, Hydrolyzed vegetable protein (12-20% MSG), Hydrolyzed plant protein, Natural Flavorings (can be called HVP), Flavorings, Kombu extract, Mei-jing, Wei-jing."

Today this list continues to grow at an alarming rate. The list in this book will be out of date in a matter of hours or days. Malted barley in bread is dangerous to your health. Malted barley is "supposed" to be fermented. If it were fermented correctly, it would be beneficial to our health. My guess is that the Food Manufacturers use chemicals to ferment the barley quicker to save time. Great for their profits, but deadly for consumers to eat.

Chemical "Liver enemy" Allergies

If you have been diagnosed by your medical doctor with an allergy, that probably means they dunno what you have. Medically speaking, an allergy could be your immune system reacting to unknown chemicals in your food.

Dr. George Wootan's theory of allergy states that allergy is usually a wastebasket diagnosis. Dr. Wootan noted an important study that demonstrates this very vividly:

"In a study of 12 children with kidney disease (nephritic syndrome) six experienced a remission when their diets were changed. Three of these children had the offending foods later reintroduced, and all three suffered immediate recurrences."

George Wootan, M.D.

Different people find that they have different reactions to the same foods. One may get diarrhea and another a headache. Arthur F. Coca, M.D., in his book called, "<u>The Pulse Test,</u>" discusses food allergies being the underlying cause of many unknown illnesses.

Dr. Coca documents medical cases from his private practice where he had many successes curing "unknown" diseases."

"Consider, for example, the case of the woman who could not be exposed to the exhaust-fumes of a bus without suffering urgent colicky diarrhea; the young woman who suffered abnormal tiredness and sinusitis from the use of a certain lipstick."

Arthur F. Coca, M.D.

Theron G. Randolph, M.D., who formed the American Academy of Otolaryngic Allergy (AAOA) was considered by many to be unorthodox because of his view that chemicals in the diet were to blame for many food allergies:

"One possible explanation is that allergic reactions often cause water retention, or edema. When bellies or ankles become bloated, this is discomforting and disfiguring. But, when the brain swells, it pushes against the inflexible skull, and pain results."

Theron G. Randolph, M.D.,
<u>"An Alternative Approach to Allergies"</u>

If you want your liver to help you live and to feel better, eliminate ALL chemicals from the foods you eat.

> "Children can become hyperactive when they ingest food colorings."
> Ben F. Feingold, M.D.

Back in 1996, Dr. Feingold's quote was the final blow that jolted me to realize that ALL food chemicals must be eliminated from my diet. We have been talking about the "known" chemicals that are on the GRAS list, (generally recommended as safe) but ALL chemicals are to be viewed as very real dangerous causes to liver health problems.

My student, Ron, had allergies. He was regularly taking prescription medication that would "sometimes" work. Friends would know immediately when Ron entered the room not because they saw him come into the room, but because they could hear his sniffling into a hanky. As an encouraging husband, Ron came to my support group because he wanted to support his wife who had diabetes. (This class is now offered on my website.)

> "I wasn't going to join the class until I heard the plan. I thought it might have something for me. I'm so happy I joined because my allergies went away." Ron

In four weeks, Ron's allergies were in remission, and as a bonus--he lost six pounds. If you have allergies, don't forget to read the ingredient list on your daily vitamin. Extra copper and folic acid should never be taken. Extra copper needs to be balanced with zinc. If the balance is off, depression may be the outcome.

(Charles Pfeiffer, M.D., Ph.D.) My advice is to get off the daily vitamin and get into daily eating fresh fruits and vegetables.

> "Folic acid (as found in multi-vitamins and children's vitamins) makes allergy symptoms worse."
> Carl C. Pfeiffer, M.D., Ph.D.

Getting your vitamins from your food is essential. Man-made vitamins should be used in the laboratory where they were invented and only given to man-made people. For God-made people, let's eat His food. What a concept.

"Liver enemy" – Chemicals - Allergies - Sulfites

Dr. Alice S. Huang of the Harvard Medical School, The New England Journal of Medicine (August 23, 1984) reported that sulfites in processed foods may cause an asthmatic attack. Ingesting sulfites can cause an allergic reaction or can be deadly to the person with severe allergies. Some aliases of sulfites are:

- Potassium bisulfate
- Potassium metabisulfite
- Sodium bisulfite
- Sulfur dioxide
- Sodium sulfite
- Vegetable freshener

Sulfites are used in processing foods - like dipping raw potatoes in a sulfite solution to prevent them from becoming black. The FDA says this chemical does NOT need to be listed on the ingredient list because everyone knows that potatoes turn black after peeling them. Really? I should know that? I didn't until I did the research you are reading right now.

"Sulfur dioxide" and several forms of inorganic sulfites that release sulfur dioxide when used as food ingredients are known collectively as sulfating agents. They are marketed as "vegetable fresheners" or "potato whitening" agents and are used to eliminate bacteria, preserve freshness and brightness, prevent browning, increase storage life, and prevent spoilage of certain food products. They are also used to improve the quality or texture of finished baked goods."

"According to some studies, 5% to 10% of all asthmatics are hypersensitive to sulfating agents. They may experience reactions ranging from relatively mild to severe. Symptoms may include difficulty in breathing, flushing, hives, gastrointestinal disturbance and possible, anaphylactic shock"

Geri Harrington, a medical researcher,
"Real Food, Fake Food and Everything In Between"

Sulfites may be used for dried spices. We have no way of knowing because the FDA says "standards of identity" means it is okay to use sulfites without listing them on the product's label.
<u>How to Dry Parsley</u>:

I did a little experiment with dried parsley found in the "spice" section at the grocery store. I bought some fresh parsley at the produce stand, and let it dry on my kitchen counter in a stainless steel wire basket. In a few days, the parsley was dry and crumbly, just like store-bought. I ground them in the blender and I had homemade parsley. Very nice.

Did the parsley have the vibrant color of my store bought parsley - Nah! There I go being optimistic - - again! What kind of dried spices do I use now? You bet'cha - I dry my own or buy "organic." Growing my own parsley and other spices in pots on my patio is a very simple and satisfying experience.

All chemicals eaten in your food are foreign to your body. These chemicals may contribute to many diseases because they poison the liver. Remember, without your liver, you will not live.

<u>Intestinal Gas:</u>

Do you get gas from beans? Most people do. The reason? Beans are harder to digest and need more hydrochloric acid to digest than other foods. Also, bloating is caused by eating prepared foods. Food Manufacturers take out many nutrients that your body must continually make extra hydrochloric acid in order to digest the NON-foods.

Sometimes this "over production" results in acid-reflux disease. The longer you eat without additives, the less and less you should suffer from painful gas, bloating or acid reflux disease.

Acid reflux disease is another warning sign from your liver that you are not drinking your daily water quota each day.

Do you remember what that water quota is? For the first few weeks you will drink one quart of Dr. B's Recipe.

Animal Products, Enemy #5

<u>Milk Contributes to Osteoporosis</u>

Sound backwards to you? The media tells us we need the calcium from milk to prevent osteoporosis. I'm saying that drinking milk causes osteoporosis. Okay, hear me out. Osteoporosis is a diet-related disease. No, it's not because you need to eat calcium in your diet! First, let's establish that food-related diseases have been a part of human history for a very long time. A few examples of diet-related diseases would be:

- In the 1500's, the disease was scurvy – caused by vitamin C deficiency.

- Beriberi was caused by vitamin B1 (thiamin) deficiency.

- Rickets (weak bones) was caused by vitamin D deficiency. Vitamin D is found in daylight. Being exposed to the sun for 10 minutes each day will solve vitamin D deficiency.

As you can see, eating the right foods is foundational to health for a long time in history. Scurvy, beriberi and rickets were all caused by LACK of nutrients from fresh foods and vegetables in the diet. No, you don't need calcium supplements because osteoporosis is NOT a calcium deficiency disease. Osteoporosis is contributed to by Food Manufacturers adding estrogen to animal feed. It's not the LACK of calcium in our diets; it is the ABUNDANCE of estrogen in our food.

By the way, the FDA says that American animals are NOT given hormones. They prefer the adjective "drugs." What are the drugs? I haven't been able to find out the exact definition of the drugs used. If it is in print, I cannot find it.

I think the difference between hormones and drugs is similar to saying six of one or a half dozen of the other. I can testify that animal products caused me to have hormonal migraines. Why did I have hormonal migraines? Because my hormones were out of balance from eating too much estrogen in my food – or should I say, "drugs?"

I believe changing the words used to describe their meat from "hormones" to "drugs" is a scam on consumers. Why would they want to change the words? My theory is that the description was changed because food manufacturers can now say, a popular buzz word phrase -"no hormones" added to their meat. But, in my opinion the true reality is that the meat is the same.

When I added the balancing hormone to estrogen called "progesterone creme." If it were an unknown drug, shouldn't I have needed the drug that balances their "drugs?" Did I totally confuse you? Here's a quote that may help clear things up:

"Estrogen dominance (too much estrogen) happens to be the major metabolic illness of the latter half of the 20th century."
John R. Lee, M.D.

Estrogen dominance – eating too much estrogen from animal products is the major metabolic illness that I suffered with when I became 52. Everyone knows that farmers in America earn more money when they have fat cows to bring to market, because fat cows are good for profits. Cows in America are given hormones – excuse me – drugs to make them fat.

The same amount of feed makes cows fat for less money. Good for profits, but not good for the people who eat their meat or eat their animal products. When we eat this infected meat or eat animal products from these sick cows, pigs, etc., we get fat and feel sick. This is a contributing factor as to why Americans are fatter than in other countries around the world where these drugs are not given to their livestock for food.

Because American cows are contaminated, men and women become fat like the animals we eat. Then in our later years, we may develop osteoporosis and prostate health problems. Not only are our beef and dairy products contaminated, but our chickens and eggs are unhealthy, too.

Marcia Herman-Giddens appeared on CNN in 2002 and spoke about her seven-year study with 17,000 girls. Her research stated that our little girls are becoming women faster than our grandmothers did in the '20's and '30's.

Why? Because women make estrogen in their body fat and American women eat estrogen in their animal-product foods. Eating this infected, unbalanced meat contributes to girls becoming women faster, PMS or premenstrual syndrome with depression and crying spells, fibrocystic breasts, (lumpy breasts) clotting periods or moodiness. Women gain weight that will not come off despite a healthy lifestyle and exercise.

When women become fifty years old, they have hot flashes. The sixties bring foggy thinking and memory loss. Then if things were not bad enough, women may get osteoporosis in their sixties or seventies.

Men do not escape health problems when they eat the drug-filled food. When their body's testosterone levels start to decrease, prostate problems may begin at about age forty five or fifty. The higher testosterone levels had kept the extra estrogen in their diet balanced, but when the lower testosterone happens normally with age, the protection disappears. (Usually slow urination is one of the first symptoms, less ability to "perform" in the bedroom and sometimes depression or low mood indicate prostate health problems.

Some tips to help lower the amount of estrogen you eat in your diet: For additional reading on this subject you may want to read my book called, "Why It Hurts to be a Woman" available on Amazon and Kindle.

- Eat only organic meat as a special occasion food and in very small amounts.

- Eliminate or reduce the amount of dairy you eat to two-or-three—half-cup servings a week. Hormone-free dairy would be a better alternative. That includes: cheese, yogurt, ice cream, cottage cheese, cream cheese, whip cream, milk or any food product made from a sick cow. Eat dairy as a treat.

- Eat free-range poultry. Tyson and Gold Kist advertise that their chickens are "minimally processed" without hormones or antibiotics. The price seems to be too cheap and may be the big give away that these manufacturers are not strict with healthy practices for raising their animals. Don't eat it.

- Murray chickens taste delicious and typically have a smaller breast size that would indicate correct practices for raising their animals. The Chicken and Yellow Rice recipe uses two cups of shredded chicken for six servings. Yes, you may have meat, but eat less – much less.

- A serving of meat means 10-to-15 percent of the entire meal. (About the size of a deck of cards.)

- Eat Organic butter - sparingly ("Organic" means butter from a cow that has not received hormones or antibiotics. I hope. You hope, because when profits are at stake we should have too much hope. None of my recipes call for butter.) If you use butter, always check the ingredient labels on butter. "Natural flavor" or "flavor" seems to be a popular additive. That could be MSG a flavor-enhancing chemical that is poisonous to the health of your liver. Salt is out – don't eat it in your butter either. They bleach the salt.

- Eat wild caught fish two or three times a week.

- When you eat out, skip the meat. Restaurants use cheap, drug-filled meat and highly processed cheese.

- Eat at least one meatless meal every day. (two meatless meals each day might be better.) I love to eat a big salad every day as a vital part of the Liver Cleanse Plan.

- Eat fresh fruits & vegetables for at least one snack every day.

- Eat nuts, seeds, or whole grain breads for the other snack every day.

- Eating two snacks every day is a healthy habit for a happier liver.

- If you eat out every day for lunch while at work, this makes an easy opportunity to eat a daily salad. Just bring your own salad dressing from home. (recipe in this book.)

- If you want to contact me to make sure of a product you've found in the store is legal **OR** to add a new product to the website, please go to: http://MigrainePhD.com/contact/

Heart disease is the number one killer of men and women in the United States.

> "It's just about impossible to kill a woman
> before menopause with a heart attack,
> but after age 65 women begin to "catch up."
> John R. Lee, M.D.

Dr. Lee contributes the rise in women's heart attacks because of HRT, hormone-replacement therapy. Giving women extra estrogen and making them "estrogen dominant" contributes to heart attacks in women.

Dr. Hermsmeyer at the University of Oregon did a study using monkeys in 1997 that agrees with Dr. John R. Lee's research that he developed while having a family practice for 19 plus years.

In 1983, Columbia University and the Framingham Heart Study (William P. Castelli, American Heart Journal, 1983; 106: 1191-2000) found:

> *"men who had had heart attacks had more of the hormone estradiol than did men who were free of heart disease."*

NOTE: Estradiol is one of the female sex hormones that contribute to women's breast size. This same hormone produces breasts in men, too.

Dr. Castelli:

> "Since there was no correlation between those who had heart disease and those who did not in the usual risk factors of smoking, high blood pressure, HDL's, and cholesterol, the evidence seems to suggest the possibility that heart disease is a hormonal disorder primarily."

Why doesn't your doctor know this information? Did he sleep through this class in medical school? No, doctors are taught that estrogen is the hormone of choice because pharmaceutical companies subsidize American medical schools. Doctors are not told the whole truth about hormonal balance and proper replacement.

The pharmaceutical companies fuel this misinformation taught in medical schools because they don't want to lose their best-selling drug. What's their best-selling drug? Their best selling drug is estrogen – sold to humans and to corporate animal farming.

Nutritional balance is the key to a healthy life. Eating foods that are made by our Creator and staying clear of fabricated, processed foods may help you to avoid heart disease.

The Recipe Plan does not ask for dairy products from a sick cow or chicken. Eggs are used sparingly in the recipes, but free-range, no hormone chicken eggs are suggested. Some grocery stores sell no-hormone, free-range chicken and beef meat. These recipes are a necessity to the Liver Cleanse Plan to help revitalize your liver function.

Processed Cheese Food is an Oxymoron

What's an oxymoron? If it's jumbo shrimp, how can it be big (jumbo) and be small or shrimpy at the same time? So, which is it? Neither, it's an oxymoron. Processed cheese cannot be food if it's processed. Here's why.

<u>Bleach:</u>

Did you know that Food Manufacturers bleach your cheese? Yep, it's disguised on the label.

- Benzoyl peroxide
- Calcium sulfate

- Potassium alum

- Magnesium carbonate

The words above are just other names for bleach for your food. These unknown words are dangerous to your health because bleach is not something you want to eat. Let me ask you, would you bleach your favorite colored blouse or pants? No? Then why would anyone want to bleach their one and only stomach?

<u>Natural Cheese has food coloring in it:</u>

Nah, can't be? Think again. The Food, Drug, and Cosmetic Act specifically allow cheeses, butter, and ice cream to contain "undeclared artificial colors." No, it's not natural colors - that would make sense. Natural colors are from blue berries or strawberries in the ice cream. Why couldn't they use the red from beets for red coloring? I'm sure you already know the answer? Right? Because beet juice would be more expensive than cheap chemical coloring.

Remember: Food Manufacturers are always looking for opportunities to maximize their profits. If using chemicals will help them save a fraction of a penny per food item, they would not be good business men or women if they did not take advantage of this no-work and no-cost profit.

What would be a Food Manufacturer's motivation? If their customers complained and stopped buying their products. Yes, sales go down, but not in America. We don't complain. Americans

just look at the price and eat it. It's all about the economy. The economy of the Food Manufacturer and the economy of the consumer. What about health? Nope. Americans don't ask.
<u>Processed Milk is not food.</u>

You probably think I'm nuts calling America's "does-a-body-good" food NOT FOOD! Please hear me out. This is another theory you need to know about. Remember, there are only two categories of food:

1) God's Whole Food.

2) Man's Processed Food.

Simple nutritional guidelines. Yes, when milk is from a sick cow and cannot be healthy because of the hormones and antibiotics, but there's more bad news about milk that renders it poison to your liver and to your health. Milk is pasteurized and homogenized, and therefore overly processed by man and rendered as a poison.

Let's investigate the processing of milk. Pasteurization is a process used to kill bacteria and prevent diseases from being transferred in the milk, right? Yes, pasteurization kills germs. No, it's not the best for the milk because nutrients are lost. It's okay and necessary to protect consumers from Food Manufacturers who are not practicing safe, clean milk processing.

In the 19th century, contaminated milk caused tuberculosis and typhoid. (Turner) If pasteurization were the only process our milk had done to it and the cows were free from drugs, it would be okay food. However, there's another process – it's called ultra pasteurization or UHT.

This process extends the shelf life of the milk. That's good for the Food Manufacturers, but it is not good for the person wanting the milk to do their body good. Why? Because the over processing of UHT takes away any food value that the milk might have had.

Lastly, homogenized milk preheats the milk (that's okay) and then forces in under 500-to-2,500 pounds of pressure per square inch, through a mesh that breaks up the natural fat globules in the raw milk.

Now, your milk does a body bad after it has been homogenized. Why? Because now the milk is no longer "natural" to the human body because these man-made tiny fat globules are so small that they can pass into the human body in places God never intended for milk to travel. The result: milk is poisonous food and will hurt your health.

Most people are not allergic to strawberries, but through the journey of eating food products from animals that have been given antibiotics, taking prescription antibiotics themselves, or certain medications to help their allergies, more allergies may develop.

Anti - means "against;" biotic - means "life." Antibiotics are against life, and kill all of the friendly germs in your body. **These friendly germs are responsible for**:

1. Making some of your B-vitamins in your gut. You have a vitamin factory right in your body.

2. Keeping the gut balanced to improve constipation or prevent diarrhea.

3. Prevents any toxic gases from the gut to back up and your liver. This promotes a happier attitude.

4. More prone to develop allergies because the good germs in the gut cannot identify a germ that will hurt you from knowing your own cells.

When the "ecosystem" of the body is not balanced with good germs and bad germs, we develop allergies. Beneficial bacteria help break down the body's waste. The healthy body has enough bacteria in their body to fill up a soup can. Subtract the bacteria which live in the gut, and the rest could all hide in a thimble. (Allison)

The immune system of an allergic person needs a chance to "sort" self and enemy out. Because of unbalanced eating, people may develop a confused immune system. A confused immune system is an immune system that is NOT working. After eating unprocessed, whole foods for several months, my student, Barbara's immune system had the opportunity to "sort" things out.

"I always thought I was allergic to whole wheat, but after a few months eating from this Liver Cleanse Plan, wheat doesn't bother me anymore." Barbara

Real Life Story::

My student Mary Elizabeth (not the same Mary who suffered with Fatty Liver Disease) was 75 when I met her. She suffered from pain in her chest. She had 18 medical appointments to seek help for the pain in her chest in one month. The pain was severe and shot across her chest; her heart would sometimes flutter, pound and skip beats. She was scared to death of just dropping dead. Her daughter suggested that she come to see me before her usual check up with the cardiologist.

When Mary Elizabeth came in for a consultation, I was so impressed as she told me what she ate. Most of her diet was whole, fresh foods. One small problem, though, she ate dairy four times a day because she wanted her osteoporosis to improve from getting calcium.

Mary told me, "I drink at least one gallon of milk every week." As an experiment, I suggested she take a break from dairy for just one week. We chose alternative foods. In one week she said:

"I feel wonderful. What do I tell my cardiologist? He thinks I'm sick." Mary Elizabeth

Giving up dairy with this Liver Cleanse Plan or cutting down is a big lifestyle change, but you should seriously consider this experiment with your diet. You may have success like Mary Elizabeth did.

Certified raw milk is food. "Regulations for certified milk are even stricter than those for pasteurized milk, with much more frequent testing - daily rather than monthly is required." (Harrington) Certified raw milk is healthy when it comes from a hormone-free cow.

"Liver enemy" - Animal Products - Allergies

Your immune system uses white blood cells to gobble up impurities in your body. These cells are called macrophages. (literally means, "big eaters." Macrophages travel in the mucus of your body for easy transporting to different parts of the body. Eating too much processed dairy may cause excess mucus in your body. If the body has too much mucus - because of eating too much processed dairy--your immune system is slowed to a stand still or to a screeching halt.

In addition, cows are given antibiotics. No, the cows are not sick. It is more profitable to farmers if their livestock keeps producing milk. If cows become sick, production is interrupted and that costs the farmer valuable time doctoring the cow and money for the vet to come to the farm to treat the cows. An easier and cheaper solution is to feed antibiotics to the cows all the time.

Antibiotics serve as a type of cheap insurance that livestock do not become ill and has a great money-making side effect that contributes to the animals gaining weight while taking the antibiotics. Unfortunately, when we eat the dairy products from these animals, we eat the antibiotics and get fat like the cows do while becoming antibiotic resistant.

Eating dairy products from a health food store can help with the transition. Please remember there aren't any guidelines to determine a "hormone-free" cow. We don't know how long the "hormone-free" cow has been free of hormones. Since birth? One month ago? Two months ago?

How long does it take for a cow's liver to get rid of all of the hormones out of their body? We don't know. Moderation is the key when eating dairy products - even from the health food store. Let dairy become a treat and not a way of life.

Calcium supplements. Good or bad?

Bad. If scientists knew the correct vitamin and mineral ratios to build strong bones, just give every woman a convenient pill. Right? The disease would be wiped out in a few years. Great? Not quite, this walking chemistry set - our body - is complicated.

Did you know that if a person's hormones are not balanced then their body won't be "signaled" to make new bone even if all the right vitamins and minerals are circulating in their blood stream? Yes, that's true, according to John R. Lee, M.D.

There isn't any magic vitamin supplement on the market with the exact combinations and ratios to make new bone in the human body, because no one knows the exact vitamin and mineral combinations. Health professionals suggest calcium and hope for the best.

"Osteoporosis is NOT caused by a calcium deficiency."
John R. Lee, M.D.

When you take calcium pills to prevent osteoporosis, it is like asking me to make bread with water and nothing else. It just can't be done. Taking vitamins is a good theory, but if your body does not assimilate (use) them, vitamins are worthless and may clog your body. Vitamins are unbalanced - only your Creator knows the right balance.

If you want the perfect calcium and mineral mix, get it from your food. Try horsetail tea because it is high in calcium. Alternatively, unsulphered, black strap molasses is high in B-vitamins and calcium.

All dark green, leafy vegetables have calcium. God's food is already balanced. God made you. God made your food. What a concept! Eat Designer foods, today.

If you suffer from muscle twitches or spasms (otherwise known as a Charlie horse,) your body may be warning you about a magnesium deficiency that may be caused from eating calcium pills. (Also, a Charlie horse may be caused by not drinking enough filtered water without fluoride and unrefined salt. Celtic Sea Salt helps your muscles and your bones.)

How do you get magnesium in your diet? No, not from a pill. A pill is unbalanced. Eat broccoli and spinach: they are excellent sources of magnesium. These balanced foods keep your body in balance.

Stop eating calcium supplements or foods that have been processed with extra calcium – like orange juice. If it's man-made calcium, it's unbalanced calcium.

Dr. Russell Blaylock cites this case study:

"The Mysterious Case of the Sick Football Players"

". . the boy's coach became concerned because of their frequent complaints of leg cramps, so he gave them a supplement of calcium. It was a hot south Florida day and the boys were playing very hard. Soon, after half-time eleven of the boys became disoriented and had difficulty walking.

The coach noticed that their speech was slurred, they complained of muscle spasms, and were breathing very deeply. Within an hour, eight of the players fell to the ground and had a full blown seizure. Two of the boys had repeated seizures. . thirteen other players reported headaches, blurred vision, muscle twitching, nausea, and weakness. Eventually all of the boys recovered."

What happened that caused this horrible incident? Dr. Blaylock summed up:

"Since they were already magnesium deficient, the additional magnesium lost precipitated this "crisis."...The boys were consuming a diet of fast-foods consisting mainly of carbohydrates and fats, and sodas containing phosphoric acid. Under the conditions of heat exhaustion that would occur after playing a vigorous game of football in the south Florida heat, we

can surmise that the boys' blood-brain barriers were at least temporarily and partially disrupted."

These men were eating a few things that contributed to their bodies being unbalanced:

- Calcium supplements.
- Sodas with phosphoric acid.
- Fast food with chemicals added.

This dietary combination coupled with being in the hot Florida sun and drinking sodas instead of filtered water without fluoride and salt, proved to be a deadly recipe for a very scary afternoon of football practice they won't soon forget. Eat balanced food for a balanced life.

Emotional Problems

Being tired and not having any energy is usually the first warning sign from a body's liver that it is not handling your unbalanced eating.

Emotional Warning signs:

* Tired without exertion
* Angry or crying without reason
* Not feeling refreshed after a night's rest
* Depression, indecision or confusion (brain fog)

"Most brain-fogged subjects have faulty sugar metabolism."

Carl C. Pfeiffer, M.D., Ph.D.

Eating processed, unbalanced food is a contributing factor to faulty sugar metabolism. Brain fog and indecision may sound like a very small problem; in fact, that may not sound like a food-related problem to you at all. Indecision becomes a problem only when it progresses to a point that making a decision interferes with living life. Like what?

- Indecision that keeps you up thinking at night and interrupts your regular sleep.

- It may be causing your appetite to change eating too much food or not enough.

- The indecision may cause you to have crying spells or interrupts your thinking.

Chemicals in your food may be contributing to these problems. You are not a weak-willed person without self control. When you eat balance in the food of your daily eating routine, and you will find a more balanced person in your every day self.

Edward Bach, a medical doctor in the 1930's, discovered that personality changes were some of the first symptoms to occur before his patients actually became physically ill. As a bacteriologist, he discovered that bacteria in the intestines existed in his patients who had a personality change.

When the bacteria were eliminated, the personality change diminished. Eating foreign chemicals in your diet, hormone-filled dairy and not eating a regular diet of fermented foods that are included in this book may contribute to this bacteria forming in the intestines.

The chemicals in processed foods will interfere with the chemical balance in the brain, too. Whole food gives the brain nutrients; sleep allows the body time to replenish brain chemicals called neurotransmitters that allow the human body to think.

In addition, regular exercise gives the brain oxygen. The brain weighs 1/50 of an adult's total weight, but requires 25% of all the body's oxygen for normal brain functioning.

Top 20 Prescription Drugs in America:

Of the top 20 prescription drugs, more prescriptions are prescribed for Prozac and Zoloft (anti-depressants) than for Prilosec (for acid reflux disease). To state that in a different way:

mental health problems are treated more often with prescription drugs than prescription heartburn medication. This sounds like a silent epidemic to me because heartburn seems to an everyday health problem in America.

The concept that mental health problems are treated two times more common than acid reflux disease is shocking. Depression is the most common mental health problem in the U.S. Please don't confuse clinical depression as a day or two feeling "blue" or "under the weather."

Clinical depression is characterized by extreme mood swings – from elation to severe depression or happiness to violent anger. A psychiatrist, who is a medical doctor, will diagnose depression as bipolar disorder or manic depression. Diagnosing a medical health disease is the sole responsibility of a medical doctor and NEVER a psychologist, social worker, or mental health counselor.

The disease of depression can have many faces. Depression can be coupled with insomnia, menstrual complaints, confusion, and moodiness. One of my students described his depression:

"I find myself just doing the tasks of the day so I can get to the next day. I don't smile like I used to. Before people would always ask me why I was so happy. I'm not my old happy self anymore."

"Mainstream treatment of bipolar disorder involves the use of lithium and anticonvulsive drugs, both of which are associated with negative, potentially dangerous, side effects. Anticonvulsive drugs have many side effects including nausea, distorted perception, and suppression of the immune system."

Jonathan V. Wright, M.D.

What's the best medicine for emotional health problems?

"The ideal diet should contain as much as possible of the following foods: whole grains and whole-grain bread, fresh or dried fruits, wheat germ, sprouted seeds, legumes (such as lentils, peas, chick peas, and beans.)"

Carl C. Pfeiffer, M.D., Ph.D.

Food is the best medicine to help improve emotional problems. Eating whole foods without chemicals will improve everyone's emotional and overall health. Let's examine a few case studies to demonstrate some real-life examples and what "normal" food does to contribute to abnormal emotional problems.

Case Study - Bipolar Disorder

My student, Edie, was diagnosed by a medical doctor as having bipolar disorder. That means her mood swings went from being depressed and sometimes suicidal to being elated and sometimes going to the mall all day and using her credit cards. Her usual eating menu:

"Well, we went out for breakfast and had donuts and coffee. I skipped lunch, but I ate a healthy dinner that I cooked from scratch."

"Tell me about your "healthy" meal," I asked.

"I made rice." she said.

"From a box?" I asked.

"No, from scratch in the bag--the yellow rice kind," she explained.

"Okay," I said, "Go on."

"Then I made green beans. That's healthy?" she asked.

"From a can?" I asked.

"Yes. Then I made my special sliced turkey," she bragged.

"Oh, how did you do that?" I asked.

"It's an entrée from the frozen food section at the grocery store. It has low cholesterol, no fat. That's healthy, isn't it?"

Let's examine her menu and how eating this menu may have interacted with her brain being able to function:

First, starting the day with breakfast is a necessity. Calling a donut "breakfast" is mental suicide because it is loaded with white, refined sugar and zero nutrients. Her body has been without food for approximately eight hours while she slept, and the donut gave her an immediate sugar rush for her brain to **TRY** and balance.

After her drug-filled breakfast of sugar and caffeine, her body officially thinks it is starving to death because of two things:

1) She hasn't had any nutrients since last night's dinner. (And, chances are that her prepared-food dinner was not balanced either.) Her body is trying to operate on caffeine and zero nutrients. Expecting a brain to function normally on these two deadly foods is not logical.

2) She decides to skip lunch. Without lunch, she is asking her brain to coast without any nutrients for 18 hours. She is setting the stage for an emotional upset. When she breaks down, family and friends will blame her circumstances and not her food as the contributing cause.

Meanwhile, she feels like an emotional failure because she broke down in front of her children. Is she an emotional failure? Absolutely and positively NO! That is a wrong way to think. She is guilty, however, of what most Americans fail to do – she DIDN'T plan what she was going to eat.

Healthy Hearsay says eat a meat entrée from the frozen food section of your grocery store and you are making a meal from scratch. Edie thought it was from scratch because she made it in her oven.

A healthy brain needs whole food in order to make the proper chemicals that will allow good emotional health. Good emotional health only comes from a brain that is able to balance chemicals in the brain. Giving her brain all that sugar and caffeine after an eight-hour fast from sleeping overnight was deadly.

A sure recipe for disaster. The canned veggies probably had more sugar in them and that contributed to her breaking down in front of the children. Her special meat entrée was cooked in an aluminum pan that was frozen with a chemistry set full of chemicals to keep it tasting good is another nail in her coffin towards a crying break down.

Dinner included packaged rice that she called healthy but it has a flavor-enhancing chemical called monosodium glutamate or MSG in it. Monosodium glutamate is a chemical designed specifically by Food Manufacturers to excite brain cells in order to make cheap, processed, and usually dead food taste exciting!

The rice was white and void of fiber, and the packet of yellow-rice flavorings is DEADLY to man or beast. MSG kills brain cells and may cause damage to our emotions.

"It is known that early damage to the frontal lobes of the brain can lead to arrested moral and social development. ...It also requires an ability to restrain our desires and emotions, otherwise known as self control."

Russell L. Blaylock, M.D.

That means when some of us eat MSG, we may become uninhibited, angry, or depressed, feel superior, or feel worthless. MSG is dangerous poison because it kills brain cells! If I eat MSG, I will suffer a migraine headache. Edie suffered from depression. Same poison, but a different reaction for a different person.

Edie ate canned vegetables with her dinner. Canned vegetables are okay food, but fresh is best. Edie had more than bleached salt in her vegetables, read food labels.

Her healthy turkey was not healthy. The turkey was a processed frozen entrée that added more foreign chemicals to her brain for an impossible balancing act. Even though the label on the food stated, "no fat, low cholesterol," the turkey was loaded with chemicals to keep this overly-processed meat entrée tasting great.

Food Manufacturers use aluminum cookware to prepare food. Aluminum is cheap and light weight, but may add to metal toxicity levels in the brain.

As you can see from her unbalanced diet, there is a genuine link between how she ate and how her brain balanced her emotional health. A healthy brain needs healthy food in order to make the correct chemical balance for good brain communication. The brain needs whole foods to keep a whole, emotionally equipped personality together.

It is essential for anyone with emotional problems to eat healthy, unprocessed, whole foods five times a day. If you eat healthy, but are sick or have mental problems, chances are very high that you are NOT eating as healthy as you think. Edie is a fine example of eating healthy that turned deadly.

A little information about how the brain thinks. The brain communicates using neurons. Neurons or nerves in the brain must not touch each other. (If a neuron touches another neuron, we would be in constant pain.) Between each neuron is a gap called the synapse. (pronounced: sin naps)

Chemicals in the brain allow communication impulses to jump across this gap or synapse to reach the next neuron. Without the right chemical balance:

- thinking is stopped
- thinking is short circuited
- too much jumping or firing happens as the brain attempts to send communication across the gap. The person seems nervous.

When repeated firing happens in the brain, we sometimes call this a seizure, panic attack, fit of rage or temper. For Edie, it meant an episode of depression.

There are 100,000 chemical reactions that occur in the normal brain each second. Correct firing requires huge amounts of the body's stored energy and nutrients to balance neuro-transmitters. (chemicals that carry a message between one synapse (space or gap between each neuron) to the next neuron.)

Emotional problems begin when these important brain chemicals are not balanced. How can this happen? A few possibilities:

1) The brain's chemical imbalance may contribute to brain signals not being able to jump the synapse (gap) to the next neuron. This person won't be able to think. Sometimes we call this "fogging thinking." Their eyes may look distant or they will not be able to form their sentences correctly. Confusion may happen.

2) Unbalanced chemicals may produce too much jumping to the next neuron from the imbalance of the brain's chemistry. Too much jumping or firing is sometimes called, "an epileptic seizure" or "being nervous." The chemicals that are in processed food may conflict with the chemical balance for normal brain communication.

Ben F. Feingold, M.D., who taught pediatrics at Northwestern University Medical School, and was chief of pediatrics of Cedars of Lebanon Hospital in Los Angeles in the 1930's, said:

"We do not know how chemicals affect the brain. Until we receive more facts, we really don't know what is going on in the human brain, or in the nervous system, and how chemicals, both natural and synthetic, might affect these mechanisms."

Ben F. Feingold, M.D.

Mental health problems remain a mystery to medical science. Dr. Carl C. Pfieffer took his patients off chemicals in their food and put them on a more natural, whole food diet, and had health improvement in 90% of his patients. Chemicals in foods may interact with the neuro-transmitters or chemicals that allow a healthy brain to function and think normally.

The balance between your food and the impact that it has on your emotional health has more of an impact on your health than you may think. Dr. Carl C. Pfieffer was able to take his patients with emotional illness and help over 90 percent by changing their diets to eating more whole foods.

A whole food would be any food that doesn't have a label. I encourage you to know how to read an ingredient list that is found on food products, but then I try to encourage you to NEVER eat any food that has an ingredient list label.

There isn't anyone doing the research on what the chemical additives and preservatives do to the brain, because NO ONE WANTS TO KNOW.

Why would any food processing business want to know how to go out of business? Who will fund such research? God doesn't advertise His food. Everyone knows fresh food is better than processed, man-made food. Or do they know?

If you are like I was, I never gave it a second thought that the FDA wasn't protecting me. So childlike, and so deadly.

Case Study – Hypoglycemia

Emotional health can be influenced by the amount of sugar in the blood. In my own life, I can feel a difference when I have not eaten in just a few hours after breakfast. I find myself getting upset quicker. I saw the same fluctuation in my children's personality when they were young and now I can see it in my grandson. They were normally very easy-going children, but without a snack, they became upset easier. When I would offer them some food, (like a banana) in a few minutes the crying would disappear.

Blood-sugar balance is an important factor for everyone's personality and overall health. If the blood-sugar level is over balanced, we may develop diabetes. On the other hand, if the blood-sugar level is under balanced, we may develop the disease called hypoglycemia. Both are diseases of the pancreas. Well, it used to be two diseases:

> "In 1949, the American Medical Association conferred its highest scientific award, the Distinguished Service Medal, on Dr. Seale Harris of Birmingham, Alabama, for research that led to the discovery of hypoglycemia."

However medical science made an about face 24 years later:

> "In 1973, the AMA did an astonishing turnabout and labeled hypoglycemia as a "non-disease," despite the experience of a large

segment of the medical community that hypoglycemia was the common denominator in many emotional complaints."

Emmanuel Cheraskin, M.D., D.M.D.

What happened in 24 years? Unsure. However, it changed the way medical doctors will or will NOT treat hypoglycemia. What are some symptoms of hypoglycemia? A few of the many include:

Dizziness, fainting, headaches, fatigue or exhaustion, drowsiness, muscle pains and cramps, cold hands and feet, irritability, crying spells, can't concentrate, excessive worry and anxiety, depression, forgetfulness, illogical fears, suicidal thoughts, muscle tremors, itching and crawling sensations, and gastrointestinal upsets. Hypoglycemia is a serious "non-disease."

"A typical hypoglycemia victim is, in fact, an emotional yo-yo, strung out on a chemical reaction he cannot control, with reactions so severe they frequently resemble insanity."

Emmanuel Cheraskin, M.D., D.M.D.

These emotional problems will happen when the body's blood-sugar level becomes unbalanced by eating too much enriched, white flour and sugary foods. In other words, processed foods!

> "One of the most crucial balances in the body is the blood sugar balance. Since the brain needs glucose from the blood to work properly, it is no surprise to find that hypoglycemia (hypo = low, glyc = sugar, emia = in the blood) and diabetes (high blood sugar) can result in the signs and symptoms of mental imbalance."
>
> Carl C. Pfeiffer, M.D., Ph.D.

Wow! Hypoglycemia is a big concern to anyone with emotional problems. When the sugar level drops in the blood, it can actually change a person's brain waves.

> "Brain waves of persons with low blood sugar are abnormal and that with chronic sugar starvation of the brain cells comes a fogged moral sense and distorted conceptions."
>
> E. M. Abrahamson, M.D.

If you are having emotional problems, please consider that they may be encouraged by low blood sugar. This metabolic disorder can be stopped by doing just two simple dietary changes:

1) Stop eating processed foods and switch to God's whole foods.

2) Eat five or six small meals every day.

The most important part of eating would be to never become hungry, because hunger will contribute to a drop in blood sugar levels. A drop in blood sugar becomes a dangerous health concern.

Case Study – Anxiety Attack

Annie was having anxiety attacks at school. She is a P.E. teacher and this was not typical to her lifestyle. She believed in fitness and practiced it every day. She exercised regularly, and took very good care of herself. When she came to see me it was only because her husband insisted. (His mother had come to see me and had good results. He was hoping I could help his wife as well.)

Annie's typical day's menu:

Breakfast: raisin bran cereal, skimmed milk, white toast with a tiny bit of margarine and orange juice.

Mid-morning snack: whole-wheat crackers and cheese.

Lunch was a salad with canned tuna from home and store-bought ranch dressing. She was too busy to take a break in the afternoon. So, she would skip a snack or grab a diet soda.

Dinner was at seven with her family. She heated up canned spaghetti sauce without any meat and made enriched noodles. She had a salad on the side with ranch dressing. Not bad?

Most Americans would congratulate her on a low-fat diet, eating snacks and for exercising every day with her students. Most Americans would be wrong. Let's look closer.

Breakfast for many Americans is boxed cereal. The only problem is that boxed cereal is NOT food. It is processed food. The hint is the box.

A study was done with laboratory rats to monitor their health while on a diet of eating just corn flakes. They gave one group of rats their normal diet of fresh fruits and vegetables and another group corn flakes.

In a few weeks, they noted that the group that was getting the fresh fruits and vegetables was doing very well. The group that was eating just the corn flakes was divided – part of the group was doing very poorly and a few of the rats had died, and the other part of the group was doing slightly better.

Neither group was doing as good as the fresh fruits and vegetables rat group. The study was to watch two groups - not three. Why did an unplanned third group suddenly emerge?

After further investigation, the researchers discovered that the third group of rats had accidentally been eating the cardboard packaging along with the corn flakes.

What is the moral of this story? If you want to be healthier, do not eat the corn flakes--eat the corn flake box- because it is more nutritious!

Raisin bran cereal isn't corn flakes, but it is a processed cereal. All processed cereals are not balanced food because of the sugar and other additives that are in the ingredient list of the cereal to keep them tasting good and crunchy.

White toast can cause brain waves to become abnormal. Why – it's just bread – Right? No. This bread is not healthy because it is enriched, white flour. All enriched food products cause an imbalance in blood-sugar levels to drop abnormally. A blood sugar drop may cause her brain waves to become abnormal as she becomes hypoglycemic – low sugar levels in her blood. Once Annie becomes hypoglycemic, she has an anxiety attack. It's just that easy.

> "Sweetened snack foods and drinks and white-flour products (refined carbohydrates) are the most deadly for the hypoglycemic. A normal pancreas, through its insulin production, is able to keep the body's blood-sugar levels under control and in balance. But when it is habitually assaulted by these offending foods, it panics and produces too much insulin, causing blood-sugar levels to plunge downward."
>
> Emmanuel Cheraskin, M.D., D.M.D.

Whole-wheat crackers are made with "enriched" flour and not whole wheat. The FDA allows the label to say "whole wheat," but in reality, the crackers are probably 10% whole wheat. These crackers are like eating white bread—deadly for the hypoglycemic and deadly for Annie.

Her dinner salad was good, but the store-bought ranch dressing is also loaded with too many chemicals to list. Tuna may be good. If the tuna is packed with spring water that includes vegetable broth in the ingredient list, it most likely has the chemical MSG in it.

Monosodium glutamate (MSG) can change Annie's brain chemistry. The canned spaghetti sauce has more chemicals. The enriched noodles will upset the chemistry of her blood sugar levels to become out of balance.

This case study brings to light another example of Healthy Hearsay. What she thought was good, and most Americans would have agreed, turned out to be a big contributing cause for her anxiety attack. Healthy Hearsay dictates healthy eating to be salads with low-fat, store-bought dressings and not eating red meat. It is all wrong. Unbalanced food contributes to unbalanced emotions. After our consultation, she said:

"I found out I was doing everything wrong." Annie

Case Study - Drug/Alcohol Abuse

I counseled a former addict who had been drug and alcohol free for about three months. Jennifer was enjoying her family after going through a church program for alcoholics and drugs. She had won children to come back home, she had a good job and had gotten back to church. She called me in tears because the night before she was very close to doing drugs and alcohol again.

Jennifer said, "Please help me. I don't want to go back to that old way of life."

I asked about her menu the day before.

Jennifer: "I had Fruity Pebbles for breakfast. I eat lots of sweets. I feel better after I eat that way. Then in an hour or two I have a snack, I have to eat something sweet again. Like a candy bar.

Lunch was simple - a bologna sandwich on white bread is my favorite with lots of mayo.

For dinner, we went out for chicken--Kentucky Fried." I was too tired to cook.

If we briefly examine Jennifer's diet, we find a diet of processed foods. The "Fruity Pebbles" for breakfast was a bad choice. Boxed cereal is unbalanced food. The rush of refined sugar into her blood stream is deadly for a former alcoholic.

"Sixty-to-seventy percent of all alcoholics are hypoglycemic."
Emmanuel Cheraskin, M.D., D.M.D.

Breakfast: Fruity Pebbles does not have any fruit – its first and second ingredient on the box is sugar and the rest of the ingredients are just chemicals. The coloring in the cereal is used to give its bright color will activate the nervous system according to Ben F. Feingold, M.D. This is deadly liver enemy to someone having emotional health problems.

Lunch: The bologna, as all luncheon meat, is loaded with deadly chemicals and nitrates. Nitrates are added to the meat to prevent botulism and are, by law in the United States, an additive that must be in ALL smoked and dried meats.

In Germany, they have outlawed nitrates and nitrites from their grocery store shelves since the 1950's. (Americans apparently lack good sense to cook their meat thoroughly before eating. That's why the FDA mandates this chemical be present in most of our processed and prepackaged meats.

The white bread is an unbalanced food and contributes to Jennifer's metabolic problem of hypoglycemia. The mayonnaise on the sandwich has the deadly oil of hydrogenated oil, plus the "spice" in the ingredient list could be MSG--a chemical deadly to brain chemistry and proper thinking.

Dinner: Kentucky Fried Chicken's secret ingredient is MSG. MSG kills brain cells and may contribute to chemically unbalancing her brain chemistry.

Here is another study done with laboratory rats that is shocking! At Loma Linda University in California, researchers induced a craving for alcohol in rats by feeding them a diet high in refined carbohydrates, low in vitamins, minerals, and proteins. (Does this diet sound similar to what Jennifer was eating?)

The rats were not psychologically or physically stressed; they were not raised by "mean parents," but the rats turned eagerly to drink alcohol when deprived of a fresh fruit and vegetable diet! What were their bodies searching for in their food? Nutrients. The nutrients were NOT present, so the body craved the alcohol in an effort to balance itself.

"The heaviest drinkers among the rats could be switched in and out of their alcoholic behavior by a change in diet."
Emmanuel Cheraskin, M.D., D.M.D.

Amazing! The rats were magically changed from alcoholics to good citizens – I mean rats just by changing their food. This sounds like I made up this story – doesn't it? Why don't doctors know this stuff? The bottom-line is just too simple to be the truth:

Give the body the nutrients it craves

and the yearning for alcohol disappears – naturally.

Here's an important concept. God's foods can <u>heal</u> emotional cravings. Man's processed foods can <u>create</u> emotional cravings.

"God's nutrition just makes good sense."
Jennifer

Remember, emotional problems are contributed to by an unbalanced diet of processed foods and foods that contain chemicals! All chemicals are dangerous to your emotional and liver's health.

One chemical has been linked to depression by one of my seminar participants. He told me that he traced his emotional depression to "propylene glycol" without any doubt. This chemical is found in many store-bought salad dressings on the market today. This additive caused him to become depressed for as long as two weeks at a time!

Propylene glycol is also called anti-freeze. Yup, it's in your food. Food Manufacturers will add propylene glycol because it is much cheaper than adding sugar to your food. This is just a money thing. They don't hate you. It is a business.

All chemicals in food are a possible problem to anyone who has mental health problems or just feeling tired most of the time. (Feeling unusually tired for no reason is the first symptom of a liver that is having difficulty functioning.)

A simple remedy for depression: Medical anthropologist, John Heinerman, cites a story from Utah's State Hospital in Provo, Utah about a woman who was severely depressed. The doctors tried many prescription medications. She did not respond to any of the medications.

Since this woman did not have the means to pay for her treatment at the hospital, her doctors found work for her to do in the hospital bakery while taking treatment. After just three days in the bakery, her health began to improve. After two-and-a-half weeks, she was not depressed anymore and was discharged from the hospital.

Why? The smell of the bread baking had medicinal qualities, and caused her depression to disappear. She said, "The freshly-baked loaves gave her an indescribable exhilaration of sorts."

Baking your own bread is by Design. The Great Designer who designed you in your mother's womb gave you a natural anti-depressant - bread baking. "To everything there is a purpose," even the purpose of bread baking helps a human's good mood. Processed, man-made bread has robbed us of this simple joy.

Did you know that almonds (dry roasted or plain) are a natural anti-depressant when you eat them without salt and other ingredients? God thought of everything when He created your food. What a concept - God knows what He is doing.

The brain has a filing system that uses smells. There's nothing like a smell to bring back a lost memory. Build pleasant memories for your children - bake and cook together at home.

If you can't bake or cook together every day, try building some pleasant memories on the weekends or special holidays by cooking together. My grandson, Jake, smells bread baking in a store and his mother reported that Jake said,

"Mommy, it smells like Nana's house."

Case Study - Migraines

Jay had migraines since he was 16 years old. Jay was 40 years old when I met him. To combat the daily migraine pain, Jay would take as many as 50 Tylenol a week or use about 11-to-14 Goodie Powders. Taking this much over-the-counter pain medication caused him to have terrible heartburn. In order to endure the heartburn, he regularly took antacids and popped them all day long.

<u>Jay's daily diet:</u>

Breakfast: eggs, sausage, and two cups of coffee.

Lunch: Jay is a construction worker and usually brought a brown bag lunch from home. His wife made him a sandwich with luncheon meat (topped with American cheese, lettuce, mayo, and slice of tomato) a small bag of chips, a few cookies or his favorite dessert - - a peanut butter cup.

Dinner: A large salad with Ranch dressing, smoked or BBQ meat cooked just right on his grill, with a baked potato.

<u>Let's examine Jay's menu:</u>

Breakfast: The sausage started his day with a chemical called "nitrates." This chemical contributes to migraines.

Lunch: The mayo has "spice" and hydrogenated oil in it. Spice could be MSG. MSG kills brain cells and contributes to a migraine. Hydrogenated oil is deadly to anyone who has muscle problems. The brain is a muscle and contributed to his migraine pain.

Since the human body is one giant muscle, it contributed to Jay's daily migraines. The luncheon meat has more nitrates in them. The chips, mayonnaise, and cookies all have hydrogenated oil. This fake, man-made oil is deadly to man and to beast and contributes to migraines.

The peanut butter cup has chemicals in it. No, it's not the chocolate. If the chocolate were just chocolate, there wouldn't be a problem. Most chocolate in America is a cheap chocolate and has flavoring added to make it taste good. I know a few friends that are from Europe and tell me that they despise American chocolate because of its horrible taste and would never consider eating it.

That "flavoring" could be MSG or other chemicals that enhance the flavor to make people "think" the chocolate tastes like good chocolate. It's "Poison." Yes, there is a chocolate recipe in this book! YAY!?

Dinner: To most people, this dinner sounds good and healthy. He didn't eat out at a restaurant. His wife cooked the meal at home. However, this meal added more insult to a very injury-filled day.

Ranch dressing has so many chemicals in it that it is deadly. MSG is directly connected to migraines. Look at the label; you are in for a big surprise when you TRY to read it. Store-bought and restaurant BBQ sauce should be called "chemistry set sauce."

It doesn't have much tomato, mostly "poison chemicals" and "spice" which could be more MSG.

After eating the recipes in this book, Jay was feeling better. By the end of the first week, he had not had a migraine. He was happy.

Unfortunately, the first weekend after he started eating the way I suggested, he was repairing his house and fell back into his old way of eating. By Monday he started his week with another migraine. He didn't have any doubt that his diet definitely made a difference to the amount of migraines he suffered with every day.

Jay has been eating this Liver Cleanse Plan for about two years now and he is not the same man I met earlier. Because of his faithful wife, Lisa, who makes sure all processed foods are removed from the house and never in Jay's lunch, he rarely has a migraine. He has lost over 30 pounds without trying, and he does not have migraines every day any more.

His wife, Lisa, has lost 15 pounds and has more energy than before this Liver Cleanse Plan. Their two pre-school boys have benefited because their used-to-be "normal" runny noses are gone.

Case Study – Painful Leg Cramps and Sore Feet

Jenny was 52 years old when I met her at a country/western dance. One evening she complained with me that every night after dancing, she would go to bed and be awakened by horrible leg cramps in the middle of the night that would force her to jump out of bed and start pushing her feet into the bedroom floor to find relief.

She got a little teary as she explained how she had tried taking magnesium pills because someone told her that would help. (Healthy Hearsay at work.) The vitamins didn't help. In desperation she had gone to a podiatrist, and he gave her a muscle relaxer. While the prescription medication helped a little, Jenny did not like taking any type of drugs.

Since we were at a dance, I suggested something quick that I knew would help her. I said, "Try chugging down four glasses of filtered water without fluoride every day before lunch with a pinch of Celtic Sea Salt in each glass. Then during the day, just drink filtered water without fluoride and salt with every meal and forget soda and coffee for awhile. Let's see if that helps." She said she would try anything in order to find relief from the horrible leg cramps.

The next time I saw her she reported that the leg cramps were almost gone. She had another problem with the soles of her feet and couldn't wear her dance shoes. I suggested she come in for a consultation.

Here's Jenny's food diary of what she ate in one day:

Breakfast:

Bran cereal with milk and fresh strawberries on top. Cup of decaf.

Lunch:

Tuna sandwich on toasted Health Nut bread.

She loved Crystal hot sauce on her sandwich to give it some ZING.

Snack:

Whole wheat crackers in a package.

Dinner:

Healthy choice dinner entrée. Diet soda.

Snack:

Microwave popcorn, low salt

To many people Jenny's diet may sound like a healthy diet, but there are some problems. As you can see, she was drinking decaf, and there isn't much mention of filtered water without fluoride in her list as we briefly spoke about that first time at the dance.

The decaf is deadly. Caffeine is natural to coffee. Removing the caffeine is accomplished with chemicals and is not a healthy choice. She should go back to drinking more filtered water without fluoride with the Celtic Sea Salt we had discussed at the dance.

The tuna fish – she ate one whole can which is not difficult to do - had a two-day supply of salt and without the water to balance it – it was a deadly combination. The Health Nut bread has partially hydrogenated oil that is deadly to a person's muscles. The pads of her feet were being inflamed from eating the man-made oil in the bread.

The hot sauce has simple ingredients: Cayenne pepper, vinegar and salt. The sauce has a high content of bleached salt. It doesn't taste salty in the slightest, but contributed to a diet that was high in sodium and low in water to balance out the salt. Plus the salt is bleached and should be avoided because it hurts everyone's health.

The snack crackers sounds extremely healthy, but it is loaded with more hidden salt and more of the same deadly hydrogenated oil.

The Healthy Choice entree is so full of bleached salt and too many other additives, I would need to be a chemist to tell you exactly what each chemical did to her poor feet.

The diet soda contributed to more of her feet problems by adding to more toxins in her body. A better choice is filtered water without fluoride and salt. The microwave popcorn has hydrogenated oil and the low salt variety is filled with more chemicals to make up for the lack of taste.

Jenny was shocked when I finished my explanation of her food diary, and said "I thought I was eating healthy!" I believe that this is a statement many Americans would identify with after they read this book.

When the human body has pain, it is a warning sign that toxins are stuck and cannot be removed. Detoxification is one of the reasons why drinking more water and salt seems to be the best kept secret for improved health. She bought this book for the exact guidelines for what to eat, how to drink and cook.

She may want to try massage therapy a few times a month to help with pain relief. Massage therapy will help to detoxify the body. Lastly, I suggested she stretch a little each day.

When she was in pain, I told her to add a heating pad as needed. Simply put her feet on the heating pad on medium heat before bed for about ten minutes.

I also suggested she read my book called, "Oxygen for Chronic Pain Management."

Three months later:

I saw Jenny at a dance, and she had a big smile on her face as she pointed down at her feet because she was wearing her dance shoes again. Success.

Magician in the Kitchen

I remember how the Magician in the Kitchen tradition was started. When my daughters were eight and ten years old, we went on our first camping vacation. One day we wanted to go horseback riding and the last ride was in 45 minutes. The girls said, "YAY, we can make it!"

I hated to burst their bubble and said, "We cannot go back to the campground, eat lunch, change clothes and be back here in 45 minutes! We'll go another day." Gee, whiz. . . you should have seen the look on their faces! Like I had dropped a bomb and killed their new puppy. They looked shocked and horrified!

Seeing their faces in stereo, I realized something: To them I had always been the magician who could take a meal out of a hat, so to speak.

"Okay," I said, "I'll try." Of course, I made it and we went horseback riding. They knew that. No, I don't remember what I fed them; all I do remember is their horrified faces.

You, too, can become a Magician in your Kitchen. Here is how. There are some staples that I always have on hand.

- A well-stocked freezer in the laundry room is crucial.

- How do I stock the freezer? I always cook two or sometimes three meals at once to save time.

- I love using the crock-pot a few times a week. Sometimes I put on two crock pots. I are a NUT. Didn't I warn you about that? With some planning you, too, can become a NUT!

- I home can with a home canner.
- I double recipes and bake once a week for freezing.

Today, my life is worth living again. I have renewed energy. My sense of humor is back. I don't ask anyone to "shoot me" anymore. (And, folks, I really meant it when I had a migraine! The pain was severe. It was the only answer I would give when my children innocently asked, "What can we do to help?" My answer? "Shoot me!")

Home canning is wonderful. It has afforded me many lazy and magical days. Freezing my soup gives me many options:
Menu:

1) Freezer or home canned soup with a tomato and cucumber salad with EVOO Salad Dressing and—— voila! Lunch or dinner is served.

2) Baked potatoes and leftover soup on top with a side salad.
Menu:

Brown rice recipe:
1) Sauté veggies in garlic EVOO is another quick way to get out of the kitchen fast. I usually make up a recipe of the Veggie Brown Rice to have on hand in the fridge. It keeps three or four days without a problem. Stir fry some veggies in garlic EVOO and

put on the rice, and maybe some of the Mock Sausage on top? I make the Mock Sausage twelve pounds at a time for freezing. A feast in minutes.

2) If I don't have any leftover rice, whole-wheat noodles boil up fast.

Menu:

Home canned red beans are another lifesaver. Heat and spoon over brown rice. Some of the Cook-Ahead Shredded Chicken on top is fantastic.

Menu:

1) The homemade deep fryer is another life jacket when you have a hungry crowd and the clock ticking. French fry onion rings are yummy.

2) Corn on the cob and French fried potatoes is my favorite. Everyone is in the kitchen waiting for the next batch while we all visit.

Menu:

1) Simple Crock Spaghetti Sauce ingredients in the crock pot the night before. (20 minutes to assemble the ingredients. Put in the fridge overnight.)

In the morning, I put the crock pot on, take out the pre-made serving-size bag of homemade mock sausage to thaw from the freezer to the fridge. When I return from a busy day, I put on the whole-wheat noodles in a pot, add the thawed and precooked meat to the crock pot, put the salad together and we eat in 45 minutes.

2) This same sauce mixture will give me a homemade pizza later in the week with the Flatbread. If I decided to home can this recipe, it makes a little over two quarts. That's a little more than two of the processed glass jars of spaghetti sauce from the grocery store.

Sometimes I fire up two crock pots. We eat one quart, and I can or freeze the other three quarts. (Am I nuts? Yup, certified.)

3) The bread dough or flatbread recipe may be used for dough into a pizza crust. When I arrive home, it takes fifteen minutes to assemble the pizza and about twenty minutes to bake until golden brown. Serve with a salad - yum.

Menu:

Salad fixing can be streamlined, too. I cut all the veggies or "fixings" and store them in a bowl with a tight-fitting lid or a gallon freezer bag. When it is time for dinner, I just assemble the salad. My bowl fixings contain: shredded or cut-up carrot, cut up broccoli, cauliflower, onion, and celery. I add lettuce to the bowl, cucumber and tomato right before serving.

Eating Out Without Being Killed

If I eat out wrong, (eating chemicals and additives in my food) I will want to **DIE**! The suggestions listed here are to help you avoid chemical-laden food in restaurants. No, you will not win friends and influence people by doing what I will suggest. In fact, you might very well be considered a "Pain-in-the-Neck Customer." Hmmmmm.

If I am at a business luncheon or special occasion where my attendance is required or may insult someone by not attending (like a family wedding.) I make sure I pre-order a steamed vegetable plate for myself.

NOTE: The food that is eaten in my house is my responsibility. God has made me the steward of my home, and I try to do the best job I know how. I try to make my home a haven in the storm for my family. If the members of your family are old enough to leave the house, they are old enough to be responsible for their own health when they are out of your stewardship.

When you eat out, notice if the menu calls a meal by a fancy name, because the food may not be food. An example would be "King Krab." The crab is probably a man-made, highly-processed fish parts and not really crab.

Vanilla-flavored ice cream is another example. The "flavor" added to the title of the food means it is not real vanilla but chemically FLAVORED vanilla ice cream. Wording is very important.

General Guidelines:

- Stay away from special sauces: they hide cheap food. Sauces are an easy place to put fake chemicals to liven up cheap food.

- The house brand salad dressing may be your best bet for food without chemicals. The house brand is usually made in their kitchen with lots of "poison." The safest salad dressing is the one you made at home and put in a bag to bring into the restaurant with you. I store my salad dressing in a baby bottle, and then put the baby bottle into a plastic baggie in case it begins to drip. Could be a mess.

- Drink filtered water without fluoride from glass NOT from plastic. The tap water is good for washing your car's body, not for putting in your body.

- Ask for steamed veggies and wild caught fish. If they don't have wild caught fish, then skip it. This is probably the safest meal in most restaurants besides a baked potato or fresh salad bar where you pick UNPROCESSED foods at the salad bar.

- French fries are normally deadly. Why? Pre-packaged French fries have probably been dipped in sulfite to keep them from turning black. No, it doesn't have to be listed on the package ingredient list. If you have allergies, don't eat French fries unless the potatoes were cut the day they were cooked by you.

- Never eat hydrogenated oil. Your server will call it by other names like vegetable oil or canola oil. The best way to judge if the oil is healthy is to ask if the oil is VIRGIN olive oil. I had a server tell me it was virgin olive oil. I believed him and woke up with a migraine.

Puh -leeze - Ask Questions: Please know this is still risky and there are no promises that this will work. Here are a few questions:

1) Was this pre-packaged or was it made on premises?

2) Does it have MSG? There are 13 other names for this deadly chemical.

3) Was it fried in vegetable oil?

4) Was it fried in margarine?

5) Was it fried in lard? (Bacon fat is okay - surprised? Because it's natural.)

6) Did you bake the potato in aluminum foil?

7) Are these real eggs or from a box or a can? In other words, processed.

8) Was the sauce prepackaged?

9) Has this beef been tenderized? (This is where Food Manufacturers inject enzymes into the live animal just before slaughter, and the tenderizer is dispersed through the animal's tissue by their own heart. Scary!)

10) Is the poultry self-basting? (Chemicals and fake fat are injected into the raw bird.)

11) Is this formed meat. (Like chicken nuggets.) Meat made from "parts." What parts? No one knows. Don't touch it.

Some nuggets are minced chicken bits, formed with the help of binders, and all sorts of other chemical additives, artificial chicken flavor and so on to make it have a shape.

Kid meals are notorious for making "cute" shapes for the meat. (Not healthy.)

12) Is the cheese processed with color additives and flavorings? Getting a straight answer to this may not be possible. Most cheese is processed in some way in America. That means making "real" cheese is a long and expensive process that most American's won't pay for because it would be too expensive.

13) Are the potatoes instant?

14) Is this fruit salad canned fruit in syrup? (In its own juice may be okay.)

15) What kind of sweetening is in your drink? Sugar is not acceptable. UNsweet tea is made with fluoride water. Man-made sugar (Aspartame, Sorbitol, etc.) is deadly and should NEVER be eaten.

If your server answers "YES" to any of the above 15 questions above, it has made their restaurant food UN-healthy for you AND dangerous to me.

What I do: My eating out technique:

Grilling my server with questions has been too stressful for me because there is a BIG risk the server, the cook and the manager does not know the answer. Will they lie? I have been lied to and waking up to a migraine has made things simpler:

1. I bring my own salad dressing from home.
2. I bring my own homemade bread and filtered water without fluoride.
3. I tip well.

Please NOTE:

I'm a cheap date. I think people like that? Are you thinking I am labeled as a NUT to my friends? Believe me, I do my best NOT to talk about my health with my friends. My family knows because I lived with them.

Are you thinking, "Doesn't anyone care that she takes homemade dressing and bread out of her purse?" If they do care, no one has ever told me or asked what I'm doing.

I do have friends at the table who ask to share my salad dressing because it smells so good, and they want to taste my bread.

The waitress or waiter doesn't seem to care what I do. I don't pour my dressing while they are bringing the food. I wait until they are gone, and I wait until the people at my table are eating and concentrating on their own food before I take out my homemade bread and dressing from my purse.

Road trips and vacations:

When I go out of town for a week, it is a challenge for me to bring healthy food for such a long time! Why? Because real food becomes bad in a few days.

Refined sugar is in everything when you eat out! Enriched flour is also in everything. Whole wheat bread at a restaurant is 10 percent whole wheat. Say what? Sorry, it's just the FDA protecting the American economy with vague food labeling. Even the fancy restaurants use chemicals in their food to cut preparation time.

Option:

Breakfast: Have a fruit salad. Finding a restaurant with a fruit bar or fruit plate on the menu is not too difficult.

Lunch and dinner: Eat a large salad with no meat, no cheese, no croutons or anything else that is man-made. Stay with fresh, raw veggies and you will have the best chance of being safe. Salad bars are good, but ask the server if they wash or soak their food with anything other than water. If they do, you are probably in the wrong restaurant.

Baked potatoes are usually fine, but ask your server if they bake their potatoes in aluminum foil. Aluminum is linked to contributing to Alzheimer's Disease because it is absorbed by the brain. The safest order choice will be the raw, steamed vegetable plate, and bring your own salad dressing from the camp ground.

Steamed Fish is usually a good choice, too. However, it should be wild caught fish. You can add lemon juice from a real lemon to the fish yourself at the table. Nothing else.

To review:

Snack:

1) Banana or other favorite fruit. (Biodegradable wrapper)

2) Self popped popcorn is a better choice than an air popper. See how to make it in your iron skillet in the recipe section.

3) Apples stay fresh well. I have even brought a whole watermelon and shared it with my relatives when I visit family. They already know I'm a NUT. All my life I have been a NUT, but today I am a certified nut or a Certified Nutritional Consultant.

4) Nuts are great. Ingredients: Pecans or Ingredients: Peanuts or Ingredients Almonds. Do you see a pattern here? Simple ingredients for feeling simply better.

What should you drink?

1) Filtered water without fluoride is best but never drink from plastic.

2) A reverse osmosis filter is good when you keep up the maintenance on the filters. Filters are a perfect place to grow mold – dark and moist. I don't trust filters. They have made me ill. The distillery removes everything from the water. It is pure. No fluoride, chlorine, parasites, viruses. Adding the Celtic sea salt will replace all the waters trace minerals.

3) When buying fruit juice, remember 100% fruit juice means no "fructose," no "flavoring," nothing but 100% fresh squeezed juice. All juices use fluoridated water and should be avoided.

My confession:

Eating out for me is too stressful. Why? Because as hard as I ask questions, read the menu several times, and tell the server exactly what I want--I still get "caught" by people that just don't understand that chemicals send me to bed for 24-to-48 hours in extreme pain. When I was young, I ate out but did not realize my headache or tired feeling was from the restaurant food. I thought I caught a bug. Remember, bugs are destroyed by your immune system. If your immune system missed a bug, you may be on the path to get cancer.

Therefore, when I'm out of town at a convention or on a vacation, I cook in my room. Shhhhh, don't broadcast that. While no one has ever told me NOT to cook in my room, I still keep my mouth closed. How do I cook for myself?

1) Quietly. I pack a one-burner hot plate, a small iron fry pan. I shop locally or bring some of the food in my carry-on luggage. I make simple meals. I like to sauté my fresh and raw foods in garlic oil or just plain EVOO. (extra virgin olive oil)

2) I make the Peppers and Rice recipe in this book, but with whole wheat small elbow macaroni instead of the brown rice. I can make the macaroni in my room, but I cannot bake the Brown Rice without an oven. There is a new trend to offer a small kitchen with an overnight stay, and that has been very nice. Look at the one-skillet recipes in this book in the Index.

3) The sauce from the Peppers and Rice recipe is so versatile as a starter recipe. I have used it with many veggie

combinations that are readily available at most local grocery store produce departments.

4) Frozen **wild** caught fish without additives seems plentiful, or I skip the meat.

5) I bring my home canned red beans and yellow rice mixture in a glass canning jar. It is heated in a small sauce pan and ready to serve. I also bring a few frozen flatbreads from home. They stay for about a week. By the time the beans are warmed on the stove, the flatbread is at room temperature and ready to stuff into a yummy burrito. I chop onion very finely to put on top. Scrumptious. A big raw salad is always easy. Fried potatoes are yummy, too.

This may sound like a pain to many people, but this is the only way I can have peace of mind that I'm not going to get sick on my vacation from chemically-processed food by eating other people's food. To me, it's worth it. Again, it is cheaper than eating out, BUT money is NOT my motivation. My motivation is PAIN. Your motivation will be to improve the health of your liver.

Recipe Section

Please use the Index at the back of this book for an alphabetical listing.

Please note: The oven is not preheated unless otherwise stated, Why? Because 1) I can't remember to preheat my oven, 2) I burn myself very easily and 3) I'm not Martha Stewart.

Homemade Deep Fryer

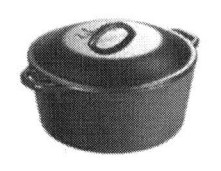

When you go to a restaurant, don't eat anything fried. Why? Because most restaurants use the cheapest oil they can purchase. (vegetable oil is dangerous to the health of your liver) The problem with cheap oil is that it is man-made and highly-processed oil. Hydrogenated oil causes many health problems.

According to Mayo Clinic, if you stop eating hydrogenated oils in your diet, you can lower your odds for having heart disease by 43%. Advice worth some serious thoughts and actions!

http://www.migrainephd.com/deep-fryer-review/

Ingredients:
One large iron pot or Dutch Oven with a lid.

You can make your own deep fryer and eat fried foods at home. The deep fryers that are on grocery store shelves are not safe. The coating peels off from inside the pot and into you. Yes, you eat it! So, try this.

What to do:
1) Buy a large iron pot with a lid. The lid cannot be a see-through lid because EVOO needs to be stored in a dark, cool place. I store my homemade deep fryer on the bottom shelf of my refrigerator, because I don't use it every day.

2) Add EVOO—extra virgin olive oil—to the pot until it is about two-inches deep. Buy a long-handled basket (not aluminum or copper, please) I prefer stainless steel. A stainless steel, slotted spoon will work, too. Always fry at a medium heat. You don't want to overheat or let EVOO smoke. That breaks down the oil and may make it UNHEALTHY.

Please note:

After 8-to-10 meals, the oil may need to be changed. If you see black on the bottom of the pot, you waited too long to change the oil.

Yes, this is a little on the pricey side, but when you've tasted your first French fry, you'll be hooked! Extra Virgin Olive Oil.

Almond Milk

Ingredients:
1 cup whole almonds (Ingredients: almonds)
2 cups of filtered water without fluoride
2-to-3 Tablespoon raw honey or Grade A Maple Syrup

What to do:
In a blender:
- **Add water and almonds**

- **Blend smooth (about 2 minutes)**

In bowl:
- **Lay a white, 100 percent cotton dishtowel over a bowl and pour in blender mixture.**

- Stain mixture by holding all four corners in one hand and squeeze the towel with the other hand so milk goes into bowl.

- Add two or three Tablespoons of honey or grade A maple syrup to your family's taste preference.

- Refrigerate and serve cold. You can use this as you would milk in any recipe.

Apple Butter

Ingredients:
9 pounds of apples (I use juicing, Red Delicious apples)
3 cups of raw honey
6 level Tablespoons of ground cinnamon
<u>Variations to Sweetness:</u>

1) Rookie version. Above 3 cups of raw honey and 6 level Tablespoons ground cinnamon for just beginning to eat this way. Wonderful for gifts.

2) Intermediate version: 2 cups of raw honey and 3 Tablespoons of ground cinnamon.

3) Master version: 1 cup of raw honey and 1 Tablespoon of ground cinnamon.

What to do:
- Core and skin apples and put into crock pot in chunks about an inch thick.

In a measuring cup:
- Stir honey and cinnamon together with a spoon.

- **Add honey combination to the peeled and cored apples in the crock pot.**//

- **Put crock pot on HIGH heat for 8 hours.**

- **Put the lid on and don't peek!**

- **After 8 hours:**

- **Stir and put on low heat.**

- **Take the lid off and allow to cook for about 8 more hours.**

- **Stir.**

Watch for the consistency you like. I like real thick apple butter. I usually cook my apple butter for a total of 16 hours. 8 hours on High with lid, and 8 hours on LOW without lid.

<u>NOTE:</u>

Since this recipe makes more apple butter than my family can eat in a month, I divide the recipe into pint jars and fill 3/4's full. I cap each jar with a canning jar lid and put in the freezer. You need head room - space at the top of the jar - so the apple butter has room to expand when it freezes. If there isn't enough room, the jar will crack.

I don't know how long this will last in the freezer because we eat it too fast. Four or five months would be my guess. Stays good in the refrigerator for three or four weeks.

Batter Mix for Frying

Ingredients:
1 cup of whole wheat flour
1-1/2 cups of filtered water without fluoride
1 large onion or bite-sized raw veggies

What to do:
In mixing bowl:
- **Add batter mix and water.**
- **Use a hand mixer to stir until smooth. This should be enough coating for one very large onion or 5 or 6 large veggies.**
- **I use my homemade deep fry with EVOO on medium heat.**

Please Note:
Do NOT cook on high heat. Smoking or burning EVOO is not good for your health.

Bean Dip

Ingredients:
4 cups of dry pinto beans
8 cups of HOT (190 degrees) filtered water without fluoride
1/2 cup garlic EVOO
2 Tablespoons chili powder .(check the ingredients on the "chili powder." If the words have any word on it that you don't understand – like flavoring? Find another brand. Organic is an excellent choice for herbs.
1 teaspoon minced onion (optional)
2 teaspoons sea salt: (See Index: Salt Example) sea salt
1/2 teaspoon cayenne pepper

Topping: 1/4 cup of dry grated goat or sheep's milk cheese

What to do:
In crock pot the night before:
- Add dry beans and HOT water.

- Let cook until morning on low heat with lid.

Next Day in iron skillet:
- Add 1/2 cup garlic EVOO or 1/2 cup EVOO with 2 teaspoons minced garlic mixed in.

- Add next five ingredients and stir well to combine all spices with Garlic EVOO.

- Add all beans and liquid from crock pot.

- Mash with fork or potato masher while cooking on low heat for about 10 minutes or until blended and mashed well. (You should see half beans, and half mashed beans in an iron skillet.)

- Slather EVOO with fingers (1/4 tsp.) in 12 X 9 baking dish:

- Transfer beans to dish.

- Pat down.

- Sprinkle dry goat's milk cheese on top.

- Bake at 350 degrees for about 10 minutes or until cheese is melted.

<u>NOTE:</u>

Serve with chips. Ingredients on the chips should say: corn and salt. The label will say "baked." These chips are still processed. Why? They should say 100% whole corn. But, they are "okay." A "Food as Medicine" choice would be: celery, carrot sticks, cucumber spears or bread for dipping instead of the chips.

This is a large recipe. I freeze half in an oven glass ware with cheese on top. This way I can take it out of the freezer, let it thaw for about four hours, and pop it into the oven at 350 degrees until the cheese is melted.

If you don't have glass oven ware to spare for storage, you can freeze in plastic. Let the dip thaw in plastic, but transfer the dip to a glass oven dish for baking.

Bread Crumbs

Ingredients:
Stale or toasted fresh bread (Made a bread oops? Bread-baking boo boos (mistakes) become bread crumbs in the blender or food processor.)

Note:
Check the ingredients on store bought bread crumbs. Please no enriched flour or partially hydrogenated oil in the bread crumbs. Those are both "Don't Touch it" foods.

What to do:
In blender or food processor:
- **Break bread apart by hand and put into blender or food processor.**

- Put on lid tightly. Pulse (start & stop blender) so blade is tossing bread around.

NOTE:

This process goes slow, and requires patience, but it is well worth the effort. I am unable to find "legal" bread crumbs that do not have "Poison" added. Poison is another word for enriched flour.

Chicken Broth - Homemade

Ingredients:
6-to-7 chicken thighs without bones (optional) and skin (not optional)
4 quarts of filtered water without fluoride
1 rounded Tablespoon minced garlic.

What to do:
Making your own homemade chicken broth is easy. Always boil enough chicken for two meals:

Some Options include: Chicken and yellow rice, Chicken Vegetable Soup, or Chicken Salad Sandwiches.

In 4 quart pot:
- **Add all the ingredients into the pot. Boil for 30-to-45 minutes. Let pot cool to room temperature.**

- **Cover and put in fridge.**

- **Next day: Skim off fat and throw away.**

Note:

I love to home can this broth for another lazy day or freeze it in a glass jar. Do not fill each jar to the top. Please give each jar an inch and a half of space of head room (air space at the top of the jar) so the broth can expand and not break your glass jar.

Chicken Broth Gravy

Ingredients:
4 cups homemade <u>chicken broth</u>
1/2 cup whole wheat flour
5-6 peeled garlic cloves
1/4 teaspoon cayenne
1/2 teaspoon sea salt: (See Index: Salt Example)
1/2 cup shredded chicken (optional)

What to do:
In blender:
- **Add broth, flour, garlic, cayenne pepper, salt**
- **Blend until smooth**

In pot:
- **Add blender ingredients.**
- **Cook until thick over medium low heat or until thick.**
- **Stir every few minutes to avoid sticking.**
- **Add 1/4 cup shredded chicken meat (optional)**

Chicken Soup Base

Ingredients:
1 cup of filtered water without fluoride
1 six-ounce can tomato paste (Ingredients: Tomatoes)
1 teaspoon sea salt (See Index: Salt Example)
1/4-to-1/2 teaspoon cayenne pepper
1 bell pepper, washed, deseeded and chopped

1 medium onion, peeled and cut
2 cups filtered water without fluoride
3 cups of homemade chicken broth
Variation:
- 1 can of beans, drained and rinsed OR home canned.

- 4 cups of veggies (Fresh or frozen - your favorites)

- 1/2 cup uncooked whole wheat macaroni

What to do:
Crock Pot Version:
In blender:

- **Add the first six ingredients and blend.**

- **Add blender ingredients to crock pot, along with the next two ingredients (Water & broth)**

- **Cook on low heat for six-to-eight hours.**

Variation:
- **One hour before you want to eat, add cooked beans, veggies and macaroni.**

- **Let cook on high in the crock-pot for one more hour.**

On the Stove, Pot Version:
- Simmer blender mixture, water & broth until they change color—about 30 minutes.

Variation:
- Add beans, veggies and macaroni.

- Cook for 30 more minutes on medium heat. (noodles will be done.)

Create a Sauce in ten minutes

Ingredients:
1 pound of tomatoes (about three medium- washed and cut core out.)
1 small onion, peeled
1/2 inch peeled, fresh ginger OR 1/4 teaspoon ground ginger
1/8-to-1/4 teaspoon cayenne pepper
1 teaspoon apple cider vinegar
1 teaspoon sea salt (See Index: Salt Example)

What to do:
In Blender:

- **Add tomatoes one at time and blend after each addition.**

- **Add onion pieces one at a time and blend after each.**

- **Add ginger, cayenne, vinegar and salt.**

- **Blend. Sauce will be smooth, but has a coarse texture.**

- **Serve at room temperature as a dip. See Idea below.**

- **Refrigerate and use within a few days. Makes 2-to-2.5 cups.**

- **Leftover Serving Idea:**

In an iron skillet:

- **Sauté veggies in garlic EVOO until tender.**

- **Add leftover brown rice, leftover salmon or other non-hormone meat.**

- **Pour over sauce from blender.**

- **Heat and serve.**

Fast and Easy Red Sauce

Ingredients:
1 medium onion (peeled)
1 Tablespoon minced garlic
1/4 cup EVOO
2 medium red bell peppers (washed, seeded & stems removed)
2 medium tomatoes (washed and core removed.)
1/2 teaspoon sea salt (See Index: Salt Example)
1/4-to-1/2 teaspoon cayenne pepper
1/2 cup whole wheat flour
Filtered water without fluoride

What to do:
In an iron skillet:
- **Fry onion, minced garlic & EVOO until tender on low- to medium heat with a lid.**

Blender:
- **Cover blades of blender with a little filtered water without fluoride.**

- **Add one at a time and blend after each: bell peppers, tomatoes, salt and cayenne pepper and flour.**

- **Pour the blender ingredients into the skillet.**

- **Simmer about 15 minutes. This will thicken the sauce, and be ready to serve over brown rice or whole wheat macaroni. (Add a pound of cooked, non-hormone meat/fish and/or a cup or two of your favorite veggie.**

NOTE: If the mixture isn't 5-to-5-1/4 cups, add more filtered water without fluoride or a small tomato to make up the difference.

French Dressing

Ingredients:
3 cored, medium tomatoes (about a half pound)
1/2 cup EVOO (Extra Virgin Olive Oil)
1/2 cup raw honey
1 stalk celery
1 Tablespoon homemade minced garlic
Pinch or 1/8 teaspoon cayenne pepper
1/2 teaspoon sea salt

What to do:
In blender:
- **Blend tomatoes (one at a time).**
- **Add EVOO, honey (more or less to your sweet preference.) and celery**
- **Blend.**
- **Add garlic, cayenne and salt.**
- **Blend.**

Makes about two cups.

Stores in the refrigerator for about two months.

Garlic Oil

Ingredients:
(NO need to be exact. The longer the garlic sits in the oil with the garlic, the more potent it becomes Very yummy)
1 head of garlic.
2 cups Extra Virgin Olive Oil (EVOO)

What to do:

- Place peeled garlic in a glass container that has a tight-fitting lid.

- Add EVOO.

- Put on lid and store in a cool, dark cabinet for at least three days before using.

EVOO Salad Dressing

Ingredients:
1/2 cup apple cider vinegar
3/4 cup EVOO (Extra Virgin Olive Oil)
1/2 teaspoon sea salt (optional)
1/2 teaspoon-to-1 Tablespoon minced garlic
1 Tablespoon fresh finely chopped parsley
　　OR 1 teaspoon dried parsley
　　OR 1 teaspoon cilantro (optional)

What to do:
- **Mix vinegar, EVOO, garlic**

- **Salt and parsley are optional.**

- **I prefer to add my salt at the table.**

* I put this in a bottle with a tight-fitting lid. You will need to shake this mixture right before pouring each serving.

Suggestion: Start with 1/2 teaspoon minced garlic and increase to 1 tsp. When I eat out, I put my dressing into a baby bottle. Then I place the baby bottle into a plastic bottle to make sure it doesn't make a mess in my purse.

Guacamole

Ingredients:
1 ripe Haas avocado, small onion and ripe tomato (see size ratio below*)
1/2 teaspoon sea salt
1/8 teaspoon cayenne pepper or a pinch or optional
1 teaspoon dried cilantro or 1/8 cup fresh, chopped cilantro (optional)
1 teaspoon apple cider vinegar

What to do:
- Peel avocado and remove seed

Blender:
- Add salt, cayenne, cilantro and vinegar.
- Add half of the onion and 1/4 of tomato
- Blend.
- Add the avocado to the blender.
- Chop the remainder of the onion and tomato quit small.
- Add to the blender ingredients that have been transferred to a bowl.
- Stir chopped ingredients gently into mixture.
- You can chill before serving or eat now.

Note:
The avocado is the same size as the tomato.
The onion is 1/2 the size of the avocado.

Variations:
- Use as a sandwich spread with a slice of lettuce. How about some tomato?

- A dip on your salad.

- I love a dollop on the side with my scrambled egg for breakfast.

Hollandaise Sauce

Ingredients:
1-1/2 cups filtered water without fluoride
1 cup peeled potatoes
1/2 cup carrots
2 Tablespoons EVOO
1/4-to-1/2 teaspoon cayenne pepper
1 teaspoon sea salt
2 Tablespoons apple cider vinegar

What to do
This recipe works better if no one sees you make it. Why? 'Cause it tastes nothing like you think it will taste. It is better NOT to know. Another "Shhhhh, recipe."

In a pot:
- Boil potatoes and carrots in filtered water without fluoride until tender. (about 20 minutes)

In a Blender:
- While still hot, pour tender carrots and potatoes and the cooking water into the blender. You may want to put a big stainless steel spoon inside to help dissipate the heat from the glass blender bowl.

- Blend until smooth.

- Add EVOO, cayenne, (I put a 1/4 teaspoon) salt and vinegar.

- Blend.

- Serve over your favorite steamed veggie. I like cauliflower and broccoli.

Hummus

Ingredients:
1 pound garbanzo beans (sometimes called "chick peas)
1/2 head peeled garlic
1 Tablespoon apple cider vinegar
1 Tablespoon EVOO (Extra Virgin Olive Oil)
1 Tablespoon sea salt
2 Tablespoons cumin
1/2-to-1 teaspoon cayenne pepper. (I use a 1/2 teaspoon.)
1 teaspoon sesame seeds (optional)
6 cups HOT filtered water without fluoride

What to do:
5.5 Quart Crock Pot:
Add the following:
- Red Beans (wash and pick out bad beans)

- Peeled garlic, apple cider vinegar, EVOO (extra virgin Olive oil, sea salt, cumin, cayenne pepper & sesame seeds (optional)

- 6 cups hot water

- Stir & cover with lid.

- Heat on low heat for 8- to-10 hours.

- Let cool with lid off for two hours.

- Puree in a food processor, blender, or wand blender. If you don't have any of these appliances, use a hand mixer.

- Because this is such a large recipe, I use pint glass canning (Mason) jars and fill them 3/4 full and freeze them. They store in the freezer for at least three months without any problems. (The time may be longer, but the hummus is eaten well before four months.)

- Serve with corn chips or on top of any meal (wraps?)

- Makes a great dipping sauce for raw veggies.

- I love this as a sandwich spread. Zips up any sandwich.

- How about hummus on top of baked potatoes? A little scallions and/or fresh cilantro is wonderful.

- get creative because hummus will surprise your taste buds as a topping.

WARNING:
If you fill the glass jars too full, they may crack. Give an inch of head room at the top. This air at the top of the jar will allow for expansion of the ingredients when it freezes.

Minced Garlic

Minced garlic strengthens your immune system, lowers blood pressure and tastes great. Store-bought minced garlic is expensive and may have chemicals added to promote a longer shelf life. Always read the ingredient label. Making your own minced garlic saves money, it doesn't have any preservatives, and it is easy for us lazy folk.

Ingredients:
1/4 cup Extra Virgin Olive Oil (EVOO) (enough to cover blades)
1 or 2 heads of garlic. (about 15-to-30 pieces, peeled)
What to do:
In a blender:
- **Add EVOO over blades.**

- **Peel one-to-two heads of garlic.**

- **Blend:(turn off and scrape sides and pulse the blender until entirely smooth.) That's it.**

NOTE: Minced garlic will store in the fridge for at least three months.

How to cut garlic

1) Put the entire head with the garlic base in the palm of your hand and push into your kitchen counter top with the heel of your hand. Cloves will separate.

2) Cut off base of a clove.

3) Cut clove in half

4) Peel should come off easily.

Mock Jelly (Raisin Spread)

Ingredients:
1 cup of raisins
1/3 cup filtered water without fluoride
What to do:
In a blender:

- 1/3 cup filtered water without fluoride

- 1 cup of raisins (Check the ingredients label. Some raisins have chemicals added.)

- Blend until smooth. Add more water if it is too thick for your preference.

- Can be stored in the fridge. Use a container that has a tight-fitting lid. Stays for about a week.

EVOO Mayonnaise

Ingredients:
1 cup apple cider vinegar
1-1/2cups EVOO (Extra Virgin Olive Oil)
1 Tablespoon homemade minced garlic
1/2 teaspoon sea salt
2 cups whole wheat flour

What to do:
Large Bowl:
- Place vinegar, EVOO, garlic and salt into the bowl.

- Add flour a little at a time and use hand mixer.

- Mixture will look thick like mayonnaise.

- Fits very nicely into a quart, glass canning jar.

- Stays in the frig for about three months.

EVOO Mustard

Ingredients:
1/2 cup Apple Cider Vinegar
1/2 Tablespoon Minced garlic
1/4 teaspoon sea salt
1/4 teaspoon turmeric
3/4 cups EVOO (Extra Virgin Olive Oil)
1 cup whole wheat flour

What to do:
Large Bowl:

- **Use a hand mixer to combine vinegar, EVOO, garlic, turmeric and salt.**

- **Add flour a little at a time and use hand mixer.**

- **Mixer ingredients will look thick like mayonnaise.**

- **Fits very nicely in a quart, glass canning jar.**

- **Stays in the frig for at least three months.**

Quick Pickles

Ingredients:
1 cup hot water
1 Tablespoon raw honey
1/2 teaspoon minced garlic
1 Tablespoon sea salt
1/4 cup apple cider vinegar
2 cucumbers (peeled & thinly sliced or cut into slices - 1/4" thick)

What to do:
In a Quart Glass Canning Jar

- Add hot water, honey, vinegar & minced garlic,
- Wash and peel raw cucumbers
- Slice cucumbers or make into spears or slices. (Your preference.)
- Put cucumbers into the hot water ingredients
- Mixture should cover cucumbers. If it doesn't, use filtered water without fluoride.
- Put on the lid and store in the refrigerator.
- Wait 24 hours and eat.

Note:
When this first batch of pickles are eaten, <u>don't throw out the juice</u>. You can make two more recipes using the same juice. Just restock more cucumbers and wait an additional 24 hours each time.

Salsa (Raw)

Ingredients:
5 medium tomatoes diced (washed and cored)
1/2 green bell pepper (washed, cored and stem removed)
2 medium chopped onions (peeled and ends taken off)
1/2 Jalapeno pepper (washed, seeds removed and chopped)
1 Tablespoon minced garlic
1 Tablespoon EVOO
1 Tablespoon cilantro
1 teaspoon sea salt (optional)

What to do:
In a Large Bowl:
- Chop tomatoes, green pepper, onions and Jalapeno.

- Add garlic, EVOO, cilantro and salt.

- Stir well to blend.

Caution!

It's best to put sandwich baggies or gloves over your hands to handle the Jalapeno pepper. Some people find the peppers irritating to their hands. (Me!) A hot pepper will be hotter if it has lines on it. The more lines, the hotter it is. A nice, green and shinny Jalapeno is not as hot.

NOTE:

Stays fresh in fridge for only a week.

Salsa (Cooked)

Ingredients:
1.5 pounds tomatoes (washed, quartered & core removed)
.5 pound onions (peeled and quartered
1 smooth jalapeño pepper (top off, seeds and ribs removed. I use baggies on my hands when I handle this pepper.)
1 teaspoon sea salt
1 peeled clove of garlic

What to do:
In a 9" x 12" glass or stainless steel baking dish:
- Add all of the above ingredients.

- **Bake at 400 degrees for one hour with a stainless steel cookie sheet on top.**

- **Allow to cool completely.**

- **Puree.**

This is a very sweet and yummy salsa.

Strained Tomatoes

Food :as Medicine: Please make the time to do this recipe because it is not made from a can and is my preferred suggestion.

Ingredients: Food as Medicine version
2-to-3 pounds of ripe tomatoes

What to do:
- **Place cleaned tomatoes into a blender and blend until smooth.**

You have few ways to remove all the skin and seeds:

1) Use a large food strainer:

- Pour the pureed tomatoes into the strainer to remove the seeds by stirring the tomatoes. The stirring action with a spoon will cause the seeds and skin to stay in the strainer.

2) Use a Food Mill:
- I have put a review of the food mill I use on my website. The food mill is pricey – about $50. But it does a faster job. You just turn the crank and the seeds and skin stay in the basket.

3) Oops method:
- One day I was trying to do my recipe from my memory. Oh, boy! I completely forgot the strainer AND the food mill method. Did I have a disaster. Nope. Tasted fine to me. You be the judge.

Fresh is best, and food as medicine. BUT, sometimes you need more options for when you don't have the time nor the energy to make the home-made strained tomato recipe.

Strained Tomatoes Okay Food Option #2

Ingredients:
- One 32 ounce can of crushed or strained tomatoes that are "legal." Legal would mean the food doesn't have any other ingredient but tomatoes. Eating from a can is NOT my first choice, but this is certainly a better choice than eating out.

- If you use tomatoes in the can that have salt added to them, then please delete the salt in the recipe. Also, be aware that Food Manufacturers change the amount of tomatoes in their product so they don't need to raise the price. I recently found strained tomatoes that were 28 ounces. So, I just added a 1/2 cup of water to make up the difference.

NOTE:
Try your best to NOT eat more than three canned goods a week is my suggestion. Why? Because canned goods are coated with a plastic inside of each can. This plastic is NOT friendly to humans and over time is leeched into the food. This plastic is called BPA or bisphenol A. Your body thinks BPA is estrogen.

Eating hormones in your food causes your body to be out of balance - the very reason why your health has escaped from your life. If you are very sick, please consider hiring someone to help you and only eat the strained tomatoes in the previous recipe until you start to feel better.

Real Life Story:
Some words on labels seem innocent, but may not be. I saw and ingredient list that said: "fresh red ripe tomatoes." I am a suspicious of the adjective "red" and would NOT buy this canned good. Red could mean anything from adding food coloring to flavor enhancers to the ingredients. Why do they mention red? Please know that Food Manufacturers are ONLY in business if you BUY their food. It is a war to them, and it should be to us consumers. If you are a confused customer, put the product gently back on the shelf, turn and . . . .RUN!

Remember, the Food Manufacturers do NOT hate you. This is just a money thing. They love your money more than they love anyone. Would you say that would be "normal?" Yeah, pretty much.

Real Life Story:
Have you ever bought a can of tuna in spring water? Sounds healthy? Right? Sure, but let me tell you a little why I may seem paranoid to you, but I'm not. Here's why. The tuna in spring water says on the ingredient list:" tuna, vegetable broth, water and

salt." YIKES . . . where did the vegetable broth come from? No mention of that on the front of the label or the "adver-teasing."

Well, the FDA allows Food Manufacturers to be vague on their food labels. Vegetable broth means the food manufacture can make up any concoction they want to add flavor to their cheap, cheap tuna. When a Food Manufacturer adds flavor, they do it with cheap chemicals that ZAP your energy. Sad, isn't it?

Vegetable Soup Base

Ingredients:
1 pound of tomatoes (about three medium- washed and core cut out.)
1/2 inch peeled, fresh ginger OR
1/4 teaspoon ground ginger
1 small onion, peeled
2 bell peppers (green or red) OR
2 Cubanelle peppers (Wash, remove stem and take out seeds of peppers.)
1/8-to-1/4 teaspoon cayenne pepper
1 can of tomato paste (6 ounce)
1 teaspoon apple cider vinegar
1 teaspoon sea salt

What to do:
In Blender:
- **Add one at a time and blend after each: tomatoes, ginger, onion, peppers, cayenne, tomato paste, vinegar and salt.**

- **Add filtered water without fluoride so ingredients are almost to the top of a 5.5 cup blender.**

To make soup:
Large glass or enamel pot.

- Add blender ingredients.

- 4 cups of bite-size fresh veggies (green beans, yellow and green squash. Usually leftovers from a week's worth of eating.)

- 1 cup shredded carrot

- 1 cup cooked kidney beans (More leftovers from my "Red Beans and Rice" recipe.)

- 1 cup Perfect Brown Rice (Again, leftovers.)

Optional:
- 1 cup leftover meat.

Hmmmm, maybe I should call this soup: "Leftover Soup?" Shhhh.

Breakfast Frittata

Ingredients:
1/8-to-1/4 cup EVOO
1/2 pound frozen French cut green beans (From 1-pound frozen bag, twist tie remainder.)
1 small onion
1 teaspoon homemade minced garlic
3-to-4 free-range chicken eggs
3 Tablespoons filtered water without fluoride
1 medium ripe tomato
1 small, peeled & chopped onion
1 teaspoon minced garlic. (about three cloves)

What to do:
Pre-heat Broiler:
In an iron skillet, on medium heat:
- Add EVOO, chopped onion, homemade minced garlic, and green beans. Fry until translucent – about ten minutes.

In a small bowl:
Beat eggs and water with a fork.

In the fry pan:
Add to fry pan and distribute evenly.
Cook on low heat until you see mixture start to bubble.
- Place sliced tomato in fry pan in a wagon-wheel design over mixture.

- Place pan under oven broiler until lightly brown. (About 5-to-7 minutes – keep a watchful eye. This goes up in smoke—fast!)

To Serve:
Use stainless steel spatula and separate from around the sides of pan. Cut into slices (like pizza) and serve.

Serves two-to-three people.

Banana Bread or Brownies (Mock)

My friends call this recipe my Brownie Recipe (Mock) because that's what they say it tastes like? Really? So, I added the Chocolate Frosting when I bring it to a Sunday covered dish luncheon. One man told me. "I love your Brownies – but what happened to the "kick?" I told him, "There's no sugar in them."

Ingredients:
1/2 cup EVOO
1/2 cup Raw Honey (use the same measuring cup. The EVOO lets the honey slide out easier)
1 free-range chicken egg (optional)
4 large bananas, peeled
1-3/4 cups of whole wheat flour or whole wheat flour
2 teaspoons of baking soda
1 cup whole, shelled pecans or your favorite nuts
Topping:
1/2 cup shelled pecans or your favorite nuts. (chopped or whole)

What to do:
In blender:
- **Add EVOO, honey, and egg into blender.**

- **Blend on low speed.**

- **Add bananas half at a time, giving blender time to catch up.**

- **Make sure the blender lid is on tight.**

- **Mixture Makes 3-1/2-to-4 cups mix or add more banana.**

- **Add the whole nuts into the blender and pulse blender a few times. If your nuts are already chopped, don't add here.**

WARNING: If you blend the nuts too long in the blender, the nuts will disappear

In large mixing bowl or pot:
- **Blend whole-wheat flour and baking soda with fork. (Put already chopped nuts in now or save for topping.)**

- **Add blender ingredients and fold into flour with a spatula. (make sure there isn't any flour on bottom of bowl.)**
- **Use your fingers to smear about a Tablespoon of EVOO on the 12" by 9" pan.**
- **Put mixture into the pan.**
- **Sprinkle about a 1/2 cup of chopped nuts on top to make it look pretty.**
- **Press the nuts in lightly.**
- **Bake at 350 degrees for 40 minutes from a cold oven with a cookie sheet on top to prevent over browning.**

My student, Sandi M,, hand mixes in one cup of raisins into the finished batter for a very tasty raisin bread. She uses a one-pound, glass loaf pan for bread.

This recipe will freeze for a month or two. I cut into serving pieces. Wrap each serving in wax paper. Then put the individual servings into a plastic freezer bag for storage in the freezer.

<u>**A great grab-and-go snack.**</u>

Banana Bread Secret:
This secret saves you money:

An over ripe banana makes the bread taste even sweeter.

Cooking ahead is the foundation of being a success eating this way. Don't forget to eat your snacks. Please take a stroll through the recipe or Index section and see if any appeal to your taste buds. This "stroll" reading some of the recipes will also serve to inspire the creative part of your brain

I'd like to hear about your new discoveries. Please visit my website and share your comments on the contact page. www.MigrainePhD.com

Chocolate Frosting

Ingredients:
2 ripe bananas
3 Tablespoons Baker's cocoa (ingredients: cocoa – nothing else - no alkali)
1 Tablespoon EVOO (extra virgin olive oil)

What to do:
In a Blender:
- **Puree peeled banana**

- **Add cocoa**

- **Puree again.**

- **Use as you would frosting.**

Carrot Cake

Ingredients:
2 cups whole wheat flour
2 teaspoons baking soda
1 teaspoon ground cinnamon
1 cup raisins

1 cup chopped pecans (or your favorite)
3 cups grated carrot (about 6 carrots)
1 cup EVOO
1 cup raw honey
1 free-range chicken egg (2 eggs makes it fluffier.)

What to do:
In a mixing bowl:
- **Add flour, baking soda, cinnamon, raisins, pecans and stir after each.**

NOTE:

Make sure the raisins are not clumping. If necessary, hand separate each raisin while in the dry mixture. Coating each raisin with the flour mixture helps to keep them separate.

- Add grated carrots and stir with a rubber spatula.
- Add EVOO, honey and egg.
- Combine. (I use a rubber spatula.)

Three Baking Variations:

Carrot Muffins

- Slather 1 Tablespoon EVOO in 12 glass muffin cups sometimes called custard cups.)
- Divide and bake at 350 degrees for 35 minutes to 45 minutes. (Toothpick will come out clean.)

Carrot Bread

- Slather 1 Tablespoon of EVOO on a one pound loaf. (Extra Virgin Olive Oil)

- Bake for 55 minutes at 350 degrees. (Toothpick will come out clean.)

Carrot Sheet Cake

- Slather One Tablespoon of EVOO on a 12" by 9" baking dish.

- Put a stainless steel cookie sheet on top. (Prevents over browning.)

- Bake at 350 for 50 minutes (Toothpick will come out clean.)

NOTE:
This recipe will freeze for a month or two. I cut into serving pieces. Wrap each serving in wax paper. Then put the individual servings into a plastic bag for storage in the freezer. A great grab-and-go snack.

French Toast

Ingredients:
4 free-range chicken eggs
Four pieces of Whole Wheat bread
1/4 teaspoon of EVOO
A sprinkle of ground cinnamon

What to do:
In a large bowl:
- Beat eggs with fork

- Slather with fingers - about 1tsp of EVOO in an iron skillet

- Dip bread into egg (front and back) and place in iron skillet on low-to-medium heat.

- Brown on one side and flip to brown on the second side.

Optional:
- Lightly sprinkle with cinnamon on one side before serving.

- Repeat with the remaining pieces of bread.

- Serve with raw honey or pure Grade A maple syrup.

Granola (Snack or Breakfast Cereal

If you are going to eat this as a breakfast cereal and need to add milk, use the Almond Milk recipe. Secondary choice: Goat's Milk, but check the ingredients.

Ingredients:
2 cups of old-fashioned oatmeal
2 cups unsalted dry roasted peanuts chopped
1 cup plain pecans chopped
1 cup plain almonds chopped
1 teaspoon ground cinnamon
3/4 cup EVOO (Extra Virgin Olive Oil)
1 cup raw honey
1 cup raisins

Note: Please check ingredients on the nuts and raisins.

What to do:
In bowl:
- Stir oatmeal, peanuts, pecans, almonds and cinnamon.

In iron skillet on low heat:
- Add EVOO & honey – let become warm

- Stir in bowl ingredients into fry pan until coated.

- Turn off heat when warm or begins to bubble.

- Slather EVOO with fingers (about a 1 tsp.) in a large baking pan.

- Spread iron skillet mixture in baking dish evenly.

- Bake at 350 degrees for six minutes.

- Stir and bake for six more minutes. (until lightly browned.)

- Let cool.

- Stir in raisins that have been separated.

NOTE:
　　Granola may be stored in a covered container in the refrigerator for at least five days. (If it lasts that long.)

Mexican Pan Bread

Ingredients:
1 medium onion, peeled 1 teaspoon minced garlic 2 Tablespoons EVOO
1 free-range chicken egg (optional)
1 can beans, drained (If you use home canned, add 1/2 teaspoon salt)

1 Tablespoon chili powder .(check the ingredients on the "chili powder." If the words have any word on it that you don't understand – like flavoring? Find another brand. Organic is an excellent choice for herbs.
1/2 teaspoon cumin
1 cup whole yellow corn flour
1-1/2 teaspoons baking soda
Optional Topping:
1/4 cup dry grated goat's cheese

What to do:
Preheat oven to 350 degrees
In iron skillet:
- **Fry onion, garlic and EVOO on medium heat until tender. Use a lid to cover. (About 5-to-10 minutes or until you can see through the onions.)**

In a blender:
- **Add egg, beans, chili powder, and cumin. .(check the ingredients on the "chili powder." If the words have any word on it that you don't understand – like flavoring? Find another brand. Organic is an excellent choice for herbs.**

- **Blend on low speed until smooth.**

In mixing bowl:
- **Mix flour and baking soda with a fork.**

- **Add blender ingredients and fold into flour mixture with rubber spatula.**

- **The onion mixture should be spread as evenly as you can over fry pan.**

- **Scrape mixing bowl ingredients evenly over onions in the fry pan.**

- Sprinkle dry goat's cheese on top. (about a 1/4 cup) Looks like Parmesan cheese (optional)

- Bake at 350 degrees for about 15 minutes.

<u>Serves four.</u>

Mock Breakfast Sausage

Ingredients:
1 teaspoon sea salt
1/2 teaspoon cayenne pepper
2 teaspoons sage OR Italian Seasoning (Ingredients are words yu recognize – like? Marjoram thyme, rosemary, savory, oregano and basil)
1/2 cup filtered water without fluoride
2 Tablespoons homemade minced garlic
3 pounds of non-hormone, free-range ground meat or grass fed beef.

What to do:
In a large bowl:
- **Combine salt, cayenne and sage.**

- **Stir with a spoon.**

- **In two-cup measuring cup:**

- **Add garlic to water and stir.**

In large bowl:
- **Add meat and mix garlic mixture into it by squeezing and mixing with your hands.**

- **Cover and let stand in the refrigerator a few hours or overnight. (This lets the spices mingle.)**

In the morning:
- Shape meat into patties and fry in an iron skillet. You may need to add some EVOO so it won't stick.

- You can fry to allow crumbling for a ground sausage look alike.

Mock Italian Sausage

Ingredients:
1 teaspoon sea salt
1-1/2 Tablespoons Italian Seasoning
1 teaspoon cayenne pepper
6 Tablespoons homemade minced garlic
1/2 cup filtered water without fluoride
3 pounds of non-hormone, free-range ground meat or grass fed beef

What to do:
In a small bowl:
- Combine salt, seasoning and cayenne.

- Blend with a spoon.

In two-cup measuring cup:
- Add garlic to water and stir until blended.

- In large bowl:

- Add meat and mix garlic mixture with spices into it by squeezing and mixing with your hands.

- Cover with plastic wrap and let stand in the refrigerator for a few hours or overnight. (This lets the spices mingle.)

In the morning:
- **Shape into patties and fry in an iron skillet like traditional sausage or break apart in the fry pan to make a crumbly ground-sausage look alike.**

Peanut Butter

I created this recipe ten years ago when all peanut butter on grocery store shelves contained deadly ingredients. The only ingredient in your peanut butter should be "peanuts." That's it. At the outside you can eat "peanuts and salt." DONE!

I once tried this recipe with raw peanuts. Boy, was I shocked when it didn't work.

Ingredients:
1 cup dry roasted peanuts
3-to-4 Tablespoons EVOO (extra virgin olive oil) MUST say "virgin"

What to do:
In a blender or food processor:
- **1-cup dry roasted peanuts, blend on low speed. (this will NOT work with raw nuts)**

- **Add 1 Tablespoon EVOO and blend. Stop adding EVOO when peanut mixture is the consistency your family enjoys. (About 3-to-4 Tablespoons of EVOO.)**

Raisin & Bran Muffins

Ingredients:
1-1/2 cups whole wheat flour
1 teaspoon baking soda
1/2 cup raisins
3/4 cup bran OR wheat germ OR old fashion oatmeal
3/4 cup filtered water without fluoride
1 free-range chicken egg (optional)
1/4 cup EVOO
1/2 cup raw honey

What to do:
Preheat oven to 400 degrees
In large mixing bowl:

- Add flour, baking soda, oatmeal and stir well. (Separate the raisins as best you can with your fingers.)

- Add filtered water without fluoride, egg, EVOO and honey.

- Stir.

- Slather with fingers 1 tsp. of EVOO into 6-to-8 glass custard cups.

- Divide mixture evenly.

- Decoration and Crunchy Protein:

- Put one teaspoon of chopped pecans or walnuts on each muffin. Then, with a spoon, lightly press into batter of each muffin. Fingers work good, too.

- Bake at 400 degrees for 20 minutes.

OPTION:

You can buy white, paper muffin liners – like you might use for cupcakes? This saves clean up time

Smoothie

Ingredients:
3 or 4 peeled banana
1 cup ice
1 Tablespoon of EVOO (extra virgin olive oil) EVOO helps to satisfy your hunger longer to the next meal.

What to do:
In a 5.5-cup blender:
- **Add peeled banana and ice.**

- **Blend until smooth.**

- **Add EVOO**

- **Drink cold.**

Any favorite peeled raw fruit should taste great for a smoothie. Get creative. I use bananas for the better half of the smoothie.

*Another option is frozen strawberries and delete the cup of ice cubes.

WARNING:
If you become sick to your stomach after drinking this Smoothie, that may be an indication of a liver in trouble. You can eat this smoothie, but decrease or eliminate the EVOO until your liver starts feeling better.

How will you know when your liver is getting better? You won't get sick to your stomach.

After Work Chili

Ingredients:
1-1/2 cups dry pinto beans
1-1/2 cups dry red beans (or whatever combo you like)
Boil 7 cups of filtered water without fluoride

Blender ingredients:
2 medium tomatoes, washed, cored and cut in half
2 medium onions peeled and cut in four
1 medium red or green bell pepper (washed and seeded)
2 Tablespoons minced garlic
1 - 12 ounce can tomato paste
Filtered water without fluoride as needed
Spices:
1 Tablespoon sea salt
1 Tablespoon cumin
1 Tablespoon cilantro
1/4-to-1/2 teaspoon cayenne pepper (I use a 1/2 teaspoon)

What to do:
In 5.5 quart Crock Pot:

The lazy secret to cooking beans in the crock pot is to use boiling water. If the water is not hot, (190 degrees) the beans won't cook to become soft.

Wash beans and pick out bad ones.

Put clean beans in Crock Pot.

Pour boiling water over beans

Cook on low heat for overnight cooking.

In 5.5 cup blender:
- Add each of the blender ingredients one at a time and blend for one or two seconds until all ingredients have been blended. Add filtered water without fluoride to make 5.5 cups. (Almost to the brim of the blender.)

NOTE:

I put a large serving spoon into the crock pot to defer some of the hot water temperature. Be careful of splashing. I don't want the blender bowl to crack from the sudden change in temperature.

- **Put on the crock pot lid.**

- **Cover and store blender bowl in the refrigerator overnight.**

- **Take out two, one-pound baggies of cooked ground meat to thaw from the freezer and put in the fridge. (Preferably non hormone)**

In the morning, before you leave for the day:
- **Rinse the beans before adding the cold blender ingredients to reduce the bean's "gas." Add 1/2-to-1 cup of filtered water without fluoride and then add cold blender ingredients.**

- **Stir well into cooked beans.**

- **Put on lid. Leave on low heat. Chili will be ready to eat after 5:00 p.m. (cook another 8-to-10 hours.)**

- **When you arrive home, add the meat.**

- **Stir and serve.**

Serving Variations:

* Serve with salad and homemade bread.

* Serve over perfect brown rice or over a baked potato

* Serve over whole wheat macaroni. I call this "Chili Mac."

Beef-broth Vegetable Soup

Ingredients:
1/4 pound organic beef tip Roast (get ready to sit down when you see the price - yes, it is worth the price!)
10 cups filtered water without fluoride
1 Tablespoon minced garlic or 1/2 head, peeled garlic
2 Tablespoons EVOO (extra virgin olive oil)
1/2 Tablespoon sea salt
1/2 pound onion, peeled
1-1/2 pounds of potatoes, peeled
2 pounds potatoes
1/2 cup diced celery (1 stalk)
1/2 pound diced carrots
1/2 pound bite-size green beans
1/2 teaspoon dried Oregano

What to do:
I start to cook this soup the night before.
In crock pot:

- **10 cups filtered water without fluoride**

- **Garlic**

- **2 Tablespoons EVOO**

- **sea salt**

- **Large onion peeled, quartered**

- **Potatoes, peeled and quartered**

- Put on low heat with the lid on for 8-to-10 hours.

In the morning:
- Use a slotted spoon to pick out the veggies, meat and peeled garlic. Put in a stainless steel pot to cool. Add 2 cups of broth to meat pot.

- Allow to cool while you cut the veggies. I broke a glass blender bowl by putting hot ingredients right from the crock pot into the blender. Sheesh!

- When you've finished all the chopping, then add cooled ingredients from the pot into the blender.

- Blend until smooth. (Add two cups or more of broth to make blending easier)

- Return blender mixture into crock pot and stir well.

- Add 2 pounds of potatoes cut into bite size pieces, chopped celery, diced carrots, green beans and oregano.

- Stir. Put on lid and let cook on low heat 8 more hours.

Serve with salad and bread.

Chicken Pasta Creole

Ingredients:
1/4 cup EVOO
1 medium onion, chopped
1 green pepper, chopped
1 teaspoon minced garlic
1 pound fresh OR frozen green beans OR your favorite veggie.
3 medium tomatoes

1/2 teaspoon cayenne pepper
1/2 teaspoon sea salt
1/2 teaspoon dried basal OR five or six fresh leaves
3 cups cooked whole wheat spirals OR elbows OR bow ties (Pick a small noodle so it will cook faster.)
2 cups of shredded cooked chicken.

What to do:
In iron skillet:
- Fry EVOO, onion, pepper, garlic and veggie on medium heat for about ten minutes until tender.

- Put noodles on to boil. Whole wheat noodles should be cooked longer than white processed noodles. (About ten minutes longer.)

In Blender:
- Add sliced tomatoes, cayenne, salt and basal.

- Blend well.

- Add to fry pan.

- Cook on medium heat for another 20 minutes or until tomatoes change color.

- Add cooked chicken. Warm.

Serve over your favorite cooked whole wheat noodles. I like elbows. Whole wheat noodles take about ten minutes longer than enriched.

Chicken and Yellow Rice

My absolute favorite recipe fo my guests. Fantastic to freeze and eat later, too. Sometimes I substitute the free-range chicken with four cups of bite-size vegetables.

Ingredients:
1 teaspoon sea salt
1 teaspoon turmeric
1/8-to-1/2 teaspoon cayenne pepper
1 Tablespoon Cilantro or Parsley
Perfect Rice Recipe
1/2 cup EVOO
1 Tablespoon minced garlic
6-to-7 cooked thigh pieces, de-boned and skinless chicken (about two cups) OR 2 chicken breasts, shredded (about two cups)
4 cups of mixed frozen or fresh veggies.
Paprika sprinkled on top

What to do:
In a small bowl:

- **Add salt, turmeric, cayenne and cilantro.**

- **Blend.**

- **Add cooked rice from the baking dish.**

- **Add mixing cup of garlic & EVOO stirred together with a spoon until blended.**

- **Use spatula to coat rice with EVOO and minced garlic mixture.**

- **Add the small bowl of spices to the rice.**

- **Mix well to evenly distribute spices over all of the cooked rice.**

- Add chicken, veggies and mix well.

- Clean the baking dish from the cooked rice recipe.

- Bake at 350 degrees for 30 minutes.

Serve with a salad and EVOO Salad Dressing.

How Hot will you go?
1/8 teaspoon for very mild

1/4 teaspoon for medium. I use a 1/4 teaspoon.

1/2 teaspoon for spicy.

Beans and Rice Casserole

Ingredients:
1/4 teaspoon red pepper seeds (Optional)
1-1/2 cups brown rice
1 Tablespoon ground cumin
2-1/2 cups filtered water without fluoride
1/2 teaspoon homemade minced garlic
2 cans beans (ingredient list: beans, water, salt – Or - One can of home canned beans (Add 1 Tablespoon EVOO)
What to do:
In a 12 by 9 inch baking pan:
- Add rice, cumin, water, garlic and beans.

- Stir

- Oven is 400 degrees

- Put cookie sheet on top. (This won't work without the cookie sheet on top. Please do NOT use aluminum foil.

- Bake for 60 minutes.

Fish and Chips

I eat sock-eye salmon because it may be the safest fish. Why? Because when Food Manufacturers try to farm (or raise) sock-eye salmon they DIE. Yup. This salmon will ONLY eat their natural diet. Smart fish.

Simply fire up the homemade deep fryer (in this book in the condiments section) for re-fried baked potatoes.

If you don't have any pre-baked potatoes, I use my food processor for thin-sliced peeled potatoes and fry crisp in my Homemade Fryer.(recipe in this book) Awesome! Crispy!

Put frozen or fresh corn on the cob in a pot and boil until done.

Wild Caught fish – no breading is needed. Fish and chips is a great recipe!

Dinner is served in stages! Everyone sits in the kitchen and visits so they are in line to get their portion of the fried potatoes as they come out hot from the fryer. Yum.

A Magician in the Kitchen Time Saver Hint:
- I bake washed potatoes and put in a 13 by 9 pan.

- Bake in the oven at 350 for 60 minutes. When they poke easily with a fork, they are done.

- Let cool. Store in a covered pan in the fridge. Ready to fry and eat.

I use as needed. Simply slice potatoes or cut into wedges. These taste insanely good and cook up in 10 minutes.

Grilled Cheese

Ingredients:
Home-made bread from this book.
Raw Milk Cheese (Homogenized dairy is dangerous to your health)
EVOO (extra virgin olive oil)

What to do:
In a skillet: (preferably iron -preheat on medium for 2 min.)

- **Add two or three tablespoons of EVOO. Place one slice of bread on EVOO.**

- **Paint EVOO on up side of both slices**

- **When bread is brown turn over**

- **Slice cheese to your liking and place on one piece of bread**

- **Put the other slice of bread with browned side down onto cheese side to make a sandwich.**

- **Brown third side of bread.**

- **Flip over sandwich**

- **Put on lid.**

- **Take skillet off heat.**

- **Set the table, get the drinks (about two minutes.)**

Makes two servings: Serve half a sandwich and homemade bowl of soup.

Jambalaya

Ingredients:
2 onions, chopped
2 Tablespoon minced garlic
1/4 cup EVOO
4 medium tomatoes (sliced, washed and cored.) about two pounds
1/8 cup filtered water without fluoride
1/4-to-1/2 teaspoon cayenne pepper
1/2 teaspoon sea salt
1 bell pepper (washed, stem & seeds removed) chopped
1/4-to-1/2 pound frozen French-cut green beans
4—Four-to five-inch wild caught flounder filets

What to do:
In iron skillet:

- **Fry onions and garlic in EVOO on low-to-medium heat until tender. (about 10-to-15 minutes.)**

- **Cook on medium heat.**

- **Wash and core tomatoes**

- **Mash tomatoes in skillet or make strained tomato recipe from this book**

- **Add fresh okra or green beans, frozen fish and bell pepper.**

- **Cover with lid and simmer 15 minutes.**

- Remove lid and break up fish with spatula into bite-sized pieces as you stir and simmer another 5-to-10 minutes.

Serve on a bed of Perfect Brown Rice and Simple Salmon compliment this recipe.

Lamb Stew

Ingredients:
1/2-to-1 pound lamb shoulder
1-1/2 pounds potatoes
1/2 pound onion
1 medium green pepper
1 teaspoon sea salt
2 pounds potatoes
3 stalks celery
1/2 pound carrots
1/2 pound beans
1-1/2 Tablespoon ground cumin

What to do:
Crock Pot (the night before)
- Add lamb

- Cut potatoes, onion and green pepper in quarters

- Add sea salt

- Add seven cups of hot water

- Cook on low heat for eight hours or overnight with the lid on the crock pot.

In the morning:

- **Drain liquid into a pot and allow veggies and lamb to cool in the crock pot during preparation of the following:**

- **Cut veggies into bite-size pieces. (potatoes, celery, carrots and beans)**

- **Strain liquid to make sure any of the bones from the lamb is in the liquid.**

- **Add the cooled veggies from the pot to the liquid.**

- **Take off all the meat from the lamb and discard fat.**

- **Puree liquid for a wonderful creamy-looking broth.**

- **Add the bite size veggies you just cut up to the broth.**

- **Add 1-1/2 Tablespoons of ground cumin and stir in.**

- **Cook with lid for another 8 hours on low heat.**

- **Add the cooked lamb shoulder a half hour before serving.**

NOTE:

If you used a lamb shoulder, don't be disappointed but this won't be much meat. The lamb is mostly for flavor and a tiny bit of meat. Shred lamb meat in a bowl and put in the refrigerator to add before serving.)

This is a large meal because I love leftovers. The rule is simple: make one-large meal for tonight, and then serve the same meal four or five days later. The extra servings are also to take to work for tomorrow's lunch.

Lazy Bread

My laziest bread recipe yet and therefore my favorite bread recipe. I love this yeast free bread. I use my counter-top slicer for thin-sliced bread that looks like normal bread. Normal means "store bought." Great for sandwiches. See the variations of ways to make this recipe look different.

Ingredients:
2 cups water
1 Tablespoon grade A maple syrup
2 Tablespoons EVOO (extra virgin olive oil)
1 Tablespoon of ACV (apple cider vinegar)
1-1/2 cups whole wheat flour

Later:
3-1/2--to- 4 cups whole wheat flour
2 teaspoons of baking soda
2 or 3 Tablespoons EVOO for coating pan

What to do in the evening:
- **My favorite way to cook is while I'm asleep. I start this lazy bread recipe during dinner or right before bed.**

In a blender:
- **Add water, ACV and maple syrup.**

- **Pulse once or twice.**

- **Add flour and put on high speed with the lid on. Stop and scrape down sides and blend.**

- **Cover with a cotton dish towel, and you are done. The recipe is gathering friendly germs from the air to** provide you with a little free yeast and friendly germs for better digestion and mood.

- The blender bowl must be out on the counter covered with a clean dish cloth for 8-to-20 hours. No, this won't hurt you, these are friendly germs free for the asking.

In the morning or sometime during the next day:
In a large kneading bowl:
- If the recipe smells good – continue. If the recipe smells bad, throw it out. Don't worry, you'll know when it is bad. I have been gathering friendly germs for over three years now, and I only had a bad smell once when I waited FOUR days. Hey...I was busy.

- Remix the blender ingredients until they turns into itself.

- Add three cups of whole wheat flour with baking soda stirred in.

- Slowly pour the blender ingredients into flour while you stir with a spoon until it becomes too difficult.

- Knead the dough with your hands into a ball.

Here's how I knead bread:
- Dredge the dough through the dry flour and fold into itself. Keep turning the dough into itself until it isn't sticky. A little sticky is fine. Add a few more Tablespoons of flour if necessary.

*A little sticky" definition:

You can form the dough into a ball and easily remove your hands from the dough without a sticky mess following you to the sink to rinse your hands off.

- **Add EVOO to a one pound glass loaf pan and use your fingers to coat bottom and all four sides.**

- **Firmly push the dough into the pan.**

- **Then remove the dough and flip it over. Now both sides of the dough have EVOO on it. Flip a third time if necessary to lightly cover the entire loaf.**

- **Let rise for one hour inside the cold oven with the door closed.**

- **Bake from a cold oven at 350 degrees for 45-to-50 minutes.**

- **Insert a tooth pick into the thickest part of the bread. The tooth pick should come out clean or bake until it does come out clean. Maybe five or ten more minutes.**

- **Cool for ten minutes and take a knife to cut around the sides of the bread or use a stainless steel spatula to pry all four sides of the bread. The bread should pop out.**

- **Slice and eat.**

Serving Suggestions:
- Try some nut butter or peanut butter on a few slices for an easy and delicious breakfast.

- Try the garlic toast for a fantastic accessory to any meal.

Think of yourself as James Bond! He looks like a regular guy, until you get to know him. That's who we are – James Bond Chefs – double naught crazy.

Please Note: I use a bread slicer for thin slices so my grandson thinks the bread looks "normal." I like to freeze it and take the bread out as needed. The bread thaws in three or four minutes or I toast it.. See "How to Freeze Flatbread" for instructions.

Lazy Bread variations

Bread Sticks

Form bread dough into long, slender bread sticks and place in a baking dish. Let rise for at least one hour and bake at 350 digress from a cold oven for about 45 minutes.

Cinnamon Buns

Disclaimer: These are NOT fluffy and flaky like what is sold at the mall. The difference? What you eat at the mall is "Face Entertainment" and NOT healthy, and this recipe is "Food as Medicine." Big health difference. This is tasty!

Ingredients to make cinnamon buns:
* ½ *of the Lazy bread recipe (NOTE: When making the bread I do NOT use ½ cup EVOO and ½ cup raw hone. Instead, I use one cup of raw honey to make this bread and no EVOO.)*

*raw honey
*ground cinnamon

Filling:
In a two cup measuring cup:
* 1 cup of raw honey
* 1 Tablespoon of ground cinnamon
* Stir with a spoon until thoroughly blended.
1 cup sliced almonds or chopped pecans
1 cup raisins (optional)

What to do:
- **Roll out bread dough with a rolling pin 1/2 inch thick. I make mine 12 inch by 15 inch rectangle. (This will fill a baking dish that is 9" by 12" leaving space for the dough to rise.)**

- **Drizzle honey and cinnamon mixture as evenly as you can on the dough rectangle.**

- **Sprinkle 3/4 cup of chopped pecans OR sliced almonds. (save the last 1/4 cup for a topping.)**

- **Sprinkle on a half cup of raisins (optional)**

- **Use your hands to roll dough from the top edge (15' side) down.**

- **Cut roll into one-inch wide pieces and put each piece into a baking dish that has been liberally slathered with 2 Tablespoons of EVOO.**

- **Place dough on the side so you see the roll of filling. 1/4-to-1/2 inch of room between each roll. Let rest for one hour.**

- Bake for 30-to-35 minutes at 350 degrees. Cinnamon buns should be golden brown. This mixture makes about 12 cinnamon buns.

IMPORTANT Note:

If you are making this recipe for guests or for your family that is used to a white sugar high, please drizzle another 1/4 cup of honey or Grade A Maple Syrup on top of the rolls immediately before serving.

Dinner Rolls or Biscuits – Bread Rolls

Ingredients:
Lazy Bread recipe:
EVOO (extra virgin olive oil) brushed on top

What to do:
- **Form bread dough into golf size balls.**

- **Place in a baking dish that has been slathered with EVOO.(slathered means to use your fingers)**

- **Brush on EVOO.**

- **Let rise at least one hour in a cold oven.**

- **Bake at 350 digress from a cold oven about 30 to 35 minutes. When they are golden brown, stick with a toothpick to make sure it's cooked to your likings on the inside. Dinner rolls are great for freezing. I wrap each roll individually in wax paper, and then in a gallon freezer bag. They last about two or three months in the freezer.**

Homemade Pizza Dough

Ingredients:
Lazy Bread recipe dough.

What to do:
- Roll out the Lazy bread dough about 1/4 inch thick and to the size of your pizza pan. I make mine in my iron skillet. A stainless steel cookie sheet with sides works well, too.
- Slather cookie sheet with EVOO and then place the dough on the pan. Cut with a knife to make the dough fit nicely.
- Allow to rest in a cold oven for one hour.
- Bake at 350 degrees for 15 minutes.
- Place all the ingredients on the crust.
- You can add Mock Italian sausage (optional)
- Black olives (ingredients: ripe olives, water and sea salt)
- Spaghetti Sauce in this book.
- ½ cup to 1 cup of goat's milk cheese sprinkled on top
- Bake at 350 degrees until the cheese is melted. (about 20 more minutes)

Pretzel Dough

Ingredients:
Lazy Bread recipe dough.
EVOO (extra virgin olive oil)

Sea salt sprinkled on each pretzel. (See Index: Salt Example)

What to do:
- **Roll out the Lazy bread dough about one-inch thick and cut into two-inch strips.**

- **Roll each strip to be round and cross at the top and tack on the side with a little water on your finger to hold two ends down.**

- **Use a basting brush to brush on EVOO.**

- **Sprinkle on some sea salt on each and lightly press into the dough.**

- **Let rest for an hour in a cold oven.**

- **Bake at 350 degrees about 30 minutes.**

Meatloaf (One Pound Grass Fed Beef)

Ingredients:
1/2 cup Whole-Grain couscous (I use one cup*)
1 teaspoon sea salt (See Index: Salt Example)
1 teaspoon EVOO
1 cup boiling hot water
1 medium onion (about 7 ounces)
8 cloves garlic (peeled)
1 pound no-hormone beef or grass fed beef
Paprika (sprinkle on top)

What to do:
In a glass measuring cup:
- **Add couscous, salt, EVOO**

- Add one cup boiling water.

- Cover & let sit for 10-to-15 minutes.

In a Blender:
- Add medium onion that has been peeled and quartered

- One entire head of garlic (peeled)

- 1 teaspoon filtered water without fluoride (optional)

In a Large Bowl:* 1 pound no hormone beef
Add measuring cup ingredients (above)

- Blender ingredients (above)

- Blend well with your hands.

- Put in glass one-pound loaf pan.

- Lightly sprinkle paprika on top.

- Bake at 400 degrees from cold oven for 45 minutes.

Serve with salad and bread.

Please note:

I use one cup of whole wheat couscous. I prefer using a higher quantity of whole grain in my food. This meat should be organic beef, or grass-fed beef. Using more whole grain extends the beef for more servings. Saves the budget a little.

You may want to build up to one cup of couscous and give your family time to adjust to the changes of less meat in their meatloaf. This meatloaf is yummy for sandwiches. Don't eat luncheon meats, they are deadly to your health.

Mexican Stir Fry

Ingredients:
1 pound of tomatoes (about three medium—washed & core cut out)
1/2 inch peeled fresh ginger OR 1/4 teaspoon ground ginger
1 small onion, peeled
1/8-to-1/4 teaspoon cayenne pepper
1 teaspoon apple cider vinegar
1 teaspoon sea salt (See Index: Salt Example)
1 teaspoon chili powder .(check the ingredients on the "chili powder." If the words have any word on it that you don't understand – like flavoring? Find another brand. Organic is an excellent choice for herbs.
1/2 teaspoon ground cumin
2 free-range chicken breasts (One package of Cook-Ahead Shredded Chicken) about 2 cups

What to do:
In blender:
- **Combine tomatoes, ginger, onion, cayenne, vinegar, salt, chili powder and ground cumin. .(check the ingredients on the "chili powder." If the words have any word on it that you don't understand – like flavoring? Find another brand. Organic is an excellent choice for herbs.**

- **Blend well.**

In an iron skillet:
- **Two cups of cooked and shredded chicken breast or mock sausage from this cookbook tastes great. If you didn't pre-cook the chicken, then add 1/4 cup EVOO to bite size pieces of chicken and fry to golden brown.**

- **Add blender ingredients as soon as chicken starts to brown.**

- Serve over whole wheat spiral noodles or Perfect Brown Rice

Pancakes

Ingredients:
In a bowl:
1.5 cups whole wheat flour
1 teaspoon baking soda
½ teaspoon sea salt (See Index: Salt Example)

In a measuring cup:
1 cup filtered water without fluoride
1 ½ teaspoon apple cider vinegar
1 Tablespoon honey or Grade A maple syrup
Extra: 1 Tablespoon EVOO for each pancake for cooking

What to do:
Preheat your iron skillet on medium heat for five minutes. I use a timer or I would burn the house down when I find myself easily distracted.
- Whisk dry ingredient together in a bowl.

In a measuring cup:
- Add water, EVOO, apple cider vinegar and maple syrup

- Stir together and then add to dry ingredients.

- Whisk together until lumps are removed. Add a Tablespoon of water to make this batter barely pour from bowl. I use a ladle.

- Add 1 Tablespoon of EVOO per pancake into the pre-heated skillet.

- Ladle the batter into the EVOO fry pan. You want a small "sizzle" to occur. I like to eat a slightly crunchy pancake. The pancake is about three-inches round.

- When you see 10 or 12 bubbles come through to the top of the pancake, it is time to flip them. Keep a watchful eye because you don't want it to burn.

- After two minutes, peek to see if the pancakes are brown on the second side before serving.

- When you make the second batch, repeat by adding more EVOO before ladling the last of the pancake batter into the skillet. This makes about six to eight small pancakes or serves about two people.

- I like making this entire batch for me. The second batch is allowed to cool and then put in a bowl with a lid for the refrigerator. The next morning, I put each pancake into the toaster to heat them up and puree some more fruit for the topping.

Home made syrup:
I puree one banana, and put into a small bowl for dipping each pancake bite. You can puree fresh strawberries or any fruit that you enjoy. Frozen fruits are NOT good unless you puree and then heat it up before serving.

Honey works good for dipping as does Grade A maple syrup.

Pasta Primavera

Ingredients:
1 pound whole wheat noodles. (I use bow tie OR linguini)
1/4 cup EVOO

2 teaspoons minced garlic
1/2 cup 100% grape juice
1/4 cup packed basil leaves OR 1 Tablespoon dried basil
1/4 Tablespoon sea salt(See Index: Salt Example)
1 small yellow onion (peeled)
1 red pepper (washed, cored and seeded)
3 small tomatoes, washed and cored
1/4 cup whole wheat flour
1 Tablespoon capers (drained)
1 six-ounce can tomato paste
Filtered water without fluoride as needed
Veggies: (4-to-6 cups thinly sliced)
1 small carrot
1 small zucchini
1 yellow squash
1 bunch broccoli florets

What to do:
- Put on noodles to boil.

In large pot:
- Heat EVOO & garlic (about three minutes on low heat.)

In blender:
- **Add grape juice, basil, salt, onion, red pepper, tomatoes, whole-wheat flour, capers, and tomato paste. (Add filtered water without fluoride or more tomatoes to make 5-1/2 cups.)**

- **Blend.**

In large pot above:
- **Add blender ingredients.**

- **Cut veggies into sticks or thinly slice: carrots, zucchini, squash and broccoli or your favorites.**

- Cook on medium-low heat with the lid on until tomato sauce changes to a deeper red color and veggies become tender. (about 35 minutes)

- Stir occasionally.

- Serve over cooked whole wheat noodles.

<u>NOTE:</u>
<u>Capers ingredients: capers, water, vinegar and salt.</u>

Peppers and Yellow Rice Casserole

See a variation in the Fry Pan Version to follow.

Ingredients:
1/4 teaspoon cayenne
1 cup brown rice
1 teaspoon turmeric
2-1/2 cups filtered water without fluoride
1/4 cup EVOO
1 Tablespoon homemade minced garlic
1 teaspoon sea salt (See Index: Salt Example)
4 cups cleaned, bite-size
6 Peppers—any kind (about one cup chopped into bite size pieces)
1 cup favorite veggie – I like corn. (frozen is good.)

What to do:
In a 12 by 9 inch baking pan:
- Add all of the ingredients.

- Stir

- Put a stainless steel cookie sheet on top.

- Bake 350 for 90 minutes.

- Serve with homemade bread and salad. Want meat? Simple Salmon in this cookbook is great.

Creative Option:

An alternative to 5 cups of cubanelle peppers, would be to put 2 cups of red bell peppers, 2 cups of green peppers and one cup of zucchini. If zucchini doesn't ring your bell, how about celery? Carrots? The four cups should be peppers—your favorite kind, and then the fifth cup can be your creative cup to make it your own dish.

Leftovers:

Breakfast: I put the leftovers in an iron skillet for 5 minutes on medium heat—until warm. Then push them over to the side, add some EVOO, and fry me an egg, Fast and easy, my two favorite words for cooking.

Peppers and Yellow Rice (Fry Pan Version)

Ingredients:
1/4 cup EVOO
1 Tablespoon <u>homemade minced garlic</u>
2 medium tomatoes, washed, cored and quartered
2 large onions, peeled and chopped
4-to-5 large Cubanelle* peppers, washed, cored, deseeded and chopped.
1 cup of filtered water without fluoride
1/4 teaspoon cayenne pepper
1 teaspoon sea salt (See Index: Salt Example)
Perfect Brown Rice Recipe
Optional Topping: Mock Sausage

What to do:
In iron skillet on medium heat:

Simmer (about 35 minutes) EVOO, garlic, tomatoes, onion and peppers until tender while you smash tomatoes.

In measuring cup:
- Add water, cayenne and sea salt.

- Stir.

- Add measuring cup ingredients into fry pan.

- Let simmer 10-to-15 more minutes.

- Serve over Perfect Brown Rice.

- Serves 4 people

- Mock Sausage topping is optional

NOTE:

Onions & peppers should be about 5-to-6 cups when thin cut. Cubanelle peppers are sometimes difficult to find. You may substitute 4-to-5 large red or green bell peppers instead. Any combination of these peppers will work. The taste is different, but great.

Shhhhhh, this is a secret!

If your children don't like the way the cooked peppers look, put their portion of the cooked mixture (minus meat & rice) into a blender. Blend into a sauce. Then let them put their "special sauce" on top of their Perfect Brown Rice. Add optional meat..

Sliced green or black olives on top are optional. Ingredients: ripe olives, water and sea salt.

Pizza Topping for 2 Pizzas

While you may cut this recipe in half for one pizza, my philosophy is that you should make both and reheat the extra pizza later in the week.

Ingredients:
3/4 cup EVOO
3 pounds of onions, peeled and sliced.
2 green peppers (optional)
Sliced Mushrooms (optional)
1 cup dry grated goat's milk cheese
Spaghetti Sauce recipe (there are two versions)
Organic Bread Dough Recipe
Mock sausage (optional)
Kitchen Sink (optional)

What to do:
In iron skillet:

- **Cook onions, peppers in EVOO on medium heat until very dark brown and soft. (about 20-to-30 minutes)**

- **On Two Cookie Sheets with an edge.**

- **Roll out dough 1/8"to 1/4" thick to the size of your pans. Use a knife to cut off the excess. I use two stainless steel cookie sheets.**

- **Bake in pre-heated oven at 360 degrees for five minutes**

- **Flip dough**

- **Generously spread onions evenly.**

- **Spoon on Spaghetti Sauce**

- Add sausage, black olives or your kitchen sink.

- Sprinkle with dry goat's milk grated cheese. This is dry cheese resembles parmesan. Key word here is cheese from a "GOAT."

- Bake for 30-to-40 minutes at 350 degrees. Cheese should be melted and crust brown.

<u>Sprinkle Mock sausage on top (optional)</u>

NOTE:
If you have kids that say, "Oooooooo, I hate onions!" Shhhhh! Don't tell them. My grandson, Jake, didn't like onions at four years old, but inhaled this pizza. The onions are very sweet and don't taste or look like "typical" onions.

Red Beans and Rice or Lazy Sunday

Ingredients:
2 cups dry red beans - 1 pound (rinsed and bad beans picked out)
7 cups of boiling hot filtered water without fluoride
1/2 teaspoon sea salt (See Index: Salt Example)
1/4 teaspoon cayenne pepper
2 Tablespoons Homemade Minced Garlic 1 Tablespoon EVOO
Perfect Brown Rice Recipe
Topping:
1 small onion, chopped (optional)
One pound of non-hormone ground meat for topping. (optional)
Or let Dad grill some chicken on the grill while the rice is baking.

What to do:
In a crock pot:
- Add the beans, hot water, salt, EVOO (extra virgin olive oil) pepper and garlic. I usually make this recipe the night

before. Make sure the water is HOT or this won't cook the beans to become soft.

- Put Crock on low heat

- Put on the lid and don't peak for about 8 hours.

In the morning:
- Turn the crock pot off or put on warm.

- Make the Perfect Rice in the oven. This takes about 60-to 80 minutes.

- Off to church or to your outing

Assemble your meal:
- Brown rice

- Red beans with a little of its juice.

- Sprinkle on some Mock Sausage. (optional) or have Dad put some chicken on the grill while the rice is baking in the oven. (If you didn't have time earlier)

- Sprinkle on chopped onion (optional)

Salmon Italian Style

Ingredients:
Wild Caught Salmon filet—about an inch thick. I like Sock Eye Salmon
EVOO Salad Dressing in this book
Paprika

What to do:
In a small glass baking dish:

- **Fresh or thawed salmon. I like sock eye salmon. Wild caught salmon is fine too. NEVER eat farm-raised fish of any kind.**

- **Liberally pour on EVOO dressing.**

- **Flip salmon so both sides are coated by EVOO Salad Dressing.**

- **Lightly sprinkle paprika on one side of the salmon.**

- **Bake salmon at 350 degrees for about 20 to 30 minutes. (depends how thick the salmon is)**

- **Salmon is ready to eat when flaky.**

Serve with EVOO veggie or a large salad and baked potato. The salad dressing is yummy poured on the baked potato, too. Back stroke! That means it is okay for your potato to swim in the salad dressing. YUM! This is food as medicine.

Salmon Patties

Ingredients:
1 can (6 ounce) skinless, boneless wild caught sock-eye salmon
(Ingredients say: pink salmon & salt)
1 free-range chicken egg
1 cup of homemade bread crumbs
1 teaspoon minced onion
1 teaspoon dried parsley

What to do:
In mixing bowl:

- Drain salmon liquid and rinse. (Can ingredients: wild caught sock-eye salmon & salt)
- Flake meat with fork.
- Add egg and breadcrumbs.
- Mix with hands or spatula to blend
- Form into small patties. (serving size)
- Fry in iron skillet on medium heat in 1/4 cup EVOO until brown. (about 15 min.)

NOTE:
 This is a kid pleaser as well as for the adult who won't normally eat fish! This doesn't taste - "fishy." The patties even taste great cold. My favorite is to pack this recipe as a snack when I'll be gone all day without time for a scheduled lunch.

Santa Fe Chicken

Ingredients:
EVOO Salad Dressing
2 non-hormone chicken breasts (One package of Cook-Ahead Shredded Chicken) about 2 cups
Salsa recipe
Red Beans & Rice recipe Perfect Brown Rice

What to do:
The night before:
- **Marinade chicken in EVOO Salad Dressing.**
- **Start red beans**

The Next Day:
- **Start the Perfect Brown Rice (takes an hour)**

- **Chicken is cooked on the BBQ - OR: fried in an iron skillet with EVOO works fine, too. Use 1/4 cup EVOO with one teaspoon minced garlic.**

NOTE:
Please no lighter fluid to start coals or any other chemicals.

Food Art:
Allow each person do layer their food the way they like. I suggest:

1) Cooked Brown Rice
2) Red beans
3) Chicken or any meat from the grill or fry pan.
4) Top with salsa (Optional)

Sloppy Joes

Ingredients:
1 large onion, peeled and finely chopped
1/2 cup EVOO (extra virgin olive oil)
1 Tablespoons minced garlic
1 pound of non-hormone meat or grass fed beef

Measuring Cup:
Add a double recipe of the strained tomatoes in this book.
2 teaspoons raw honey
1 teaspoon sea salt (See Index: Salt Example)
1/2 cup old fashioned oatmeal

What to do:
In an Iron Skillet:
- One chopped onion

- 1/2 cup EVOO (extra virgin olive oil)

- 2 Tablespoons homemade minced garlic

- Cook on medium low heat for 10 minutes.

- Onion will be soft

- Add no-hormone ground beef

- Brown (about ten minutes more)

- Add measuring cup ingredients

- Add oatmeal

- Simmer and stir for about 15 to 20 minutes until thick sauce.

- Use a lid to half cover the iron skillet.

- Serve over whole wheat bread, or whole wheat elbows or brown rice.

Spaghetti Sauce (Crock)

Ingredients:
1 lb Carrots
1/2 lb onions
1 Jalapeño peppers 2-1/2" long (optional)
1/2 head peeled garlic
1/2 cup EVOO (Extra Virgin Olive Oil)
2 cups filtered water without fluoride
1 teaspoon sea salt (See Index: Salt Example)
1 recipe of strained Tomato recipe in this book
1 tsp coriander
1 rounded Tablespoon course Oregano or 2 tsp. Fine oregano
1 pound whole wheat pasta

What to do:

In Crock Pot:
- Add cleaned carrots without tops, peeled onions cut in quarters.
- Add peppers. * (wash, seed and take tops off) optional
- Peel garlic from whole head
- 2 cups filtered water without fluoride & sea salt
- 1/2 cup EVOO
- Cover crock pot.
- On low heat for overnight. Or on high heat for four hours.
- Turn off crock pot and allow to cool.

In blender:
- **Add crock pot ingredients**
- **Mixture should be almost 5-1/2 cups. Add more water to make up the difference.**
- **Blend well. (about one minute)**

In large pot that has lid (Glass or stainless steel)

- **Pour in blender ingredients,**
- **Stir in strained tomato recipe from this book until blended.**
- **Add coriander, and oregano.**
- **Stir into sauce. Your sauce is done.**
- **Add one pound cooked whole wheat noodles. Sometimes I use spirals, spaghetti, Penn—your choice. This sauce**

freezes well. **3/4 fill a quart canning jar. Put on lid and put in freezer. Stays 3-to-6 months.**

Warning:

When freezing this sauce it is crucial to fill glass quart jars only 3/4 full. If the jar is more than 3/4's full, the glass may break.

Pizza:

I also use this sauce for pizza. Use the recipe for pizza dough. The flatbread recipe works well, too.

Spaghetti Sauce (Oven)

Ingredients:
1 lb Carrots
1/2 lb onions
1 Jalapeño peppers 2-1/2" long (optional)
1/2 head peeled garlic
1/2 cup EVOO (Extra Virgin Olive Oil)
2 cups filtered water without fluoride
1 teaspoon sea salt (See Index: Salt Example)
1 recipe of Strained Tomato recipe in this book
1 tsp coriander
1 rounded Tablespoon course Oregano or 2 tsp. Fine oregano
1 pound whole wheat pasta

What to do:
In 9 by 12 glass pan:
- **Add cleaned carrots without tops, peeled onions cut in quarters.**

- **Add peppers. * (wash, seed and take tops off) optional**

- **Peel garlic from one whole head**

- 2 cups filtered water without fluoride & sea salt

- 1/2 cup EVOO

- Place in oven at 350 degree for one hour. Veggies are soft.

- Cover pan with cookie sheet. (Stainless steel)

- Turn off oven and allow to cool.

In blender:
- Add all of baking dish ingredients

- Mixture should be almost 5-1/2 cups. Add more water to make up the difference.

- Blend well. (about one minute)

In large pot that has lid
- Pour in blender ingredients,

- Stir in strained tomatoes until blended.

- Add coriander, and oregano.

- Stir into sauce. Your sauce is done.

- Add one pound cooked whole wheat noodles. Sometimes I use spirals, spaghetti, Penn—your choice. This sauce freezes well. 3/4 fill a quart canning jar. Put on lid and put in freezer. Stays 3-to-6 months.

Warning:
When freezing this sauce it is crucial to fill glass quart jars only 3/4 full. If the jar is more than 3/4's full, the glass may break.
Pizza:

I also use this sauce for pizza. Use the recipe for pizza dough. The flatbread recipe works well, too.

Stir Fry

Ingredients:
2 small onions, peeled
1/4 cup Garlic EVOO <u>OR</u> 1 teaspoon minced garlic stirred into 1/4 cup EVOO
4 cups of your favorite fresh or frozen veggie
2 cups raw chicken breast cut into bite-size pieces
1 cup filtered water without fluoride
1/8-to-1/4 teaspoon cayenne pepper
1 teaspoon sea salt (See Index: Salt Example)
2 teaspoons mustard powder
1 rounded Tablespoon whole wheat flour
Perfect Brown Rice Recipe

What to do:
In an iron skillet:

- **Add onions, and garlic EVOO.**

- **Cook on medium heat until brown and caramel looking. (Cover for 20 minutes.)**

- **Add veggies and meat. and cook on medium heat until chicken is done. (Cover with lid and cook 20 more minutes.)**

- **In a measuring cup add: water salt, mustard powder, cayenne pepper and whole-wheat flour. Stir with spoon until blended without lumps.**

- **Add filtered water without fluoride mixture to skillet.**

- **Cook without lid for 10 minutes. Thickens slightly.**

- Serve over Perfect Brown Rice.

Stuffed Peppers

A crowd pleaser!

Ingredients:
You need two recipes:
1) <u>Fast n' Easy Red Sauce</u>
2) 1/2-to-1 recipe of cooked Perfect Brown Rice Recipe
The third recipe is optional:
1 package of frozen non-hormone ground meat.
2-1/2-to 3 cups veggies (I use: chopped celery, chopped onion, frozen corn & frozen peas.)
12 large green or red bell peppers

Topping:
Dry grated goat's milk cheese
What to do:
In a Large Bowl or Pot:
- **Mix sauce, rice, meat and veggies**

- **Wash peppers: take off the tops and de-seed. (Tops can be put into a freezer bag. Pepper tops freeze without a problem. They work well for the Fast n' Easy Red Sauce.)**

- **Stuff mixture into the raw peppers and place into a baking dish.**

- **Top with Homemade Breadcrumb Mix or grated goat's milk cheese.**

- **Bake at 350 degrees for 40-to-45 minutes. Poke with fork. When peppers are tender, they are done. Your family and guests will think you are a gourmet cook.**

Note for Stuffed Pepper:

Stuffed peppers is a crowd pleaser. When I have company at my house or when I am invited to eat at a friend's house — this is a winner! No, I cannot eat at most friends' home. Why? Well, most people think they cook from scratch, and I should be able to eat their "non-restaurant food" without getting a migraine.

One problem— most people "think" that using mayonnaise in their potato salad is scratch. Sorry, mayonnaise is not food—it's full of chemicals. Mayo gives me a health problem. How about a "homemade, scratch pie" but the crust is bought at the grocery store. Oops, again. I will have a migraine.

Then there's the famous green-bean casserole with mushroom soup and those crunchy onions on the top—migraine again. (The soup and the canned onion both have MSG.) Dijon Mustard? Nope. Worcheshire Sauce? Nope. All contain chemicals that trigger migraine and liver diseases.

Americans need to be re-programmed to the real meaning of "scratch." Advertisers have done their job well—we are all brainwashed.

Texas Fries

Ingredients:
6-to-8 medium baking potatoes
1/2-to-3/4 cup EVOO Mustard

1/4 cup of minced onion
1/2 teaspoon sea salt (See Index: Salt Example)
1/8-to-1/4 teaspoon cayenne pepper

What to do:
- Wash or scrub potatoes with a vegetable brush.

- Cut potatoes in half, and then cut halves into strips about 1/4 inch thick.

In Gallon Freezer Bag:
- Add potatoes.

- Add EVOO Mustard, minced onion, sea salt and cayenne.

- Close bag to mix by gently squeezing until mixture coats all the potatoes.

- Transfer to a 13 by 9 glass baking dish brushed of slathered with fingers with 1/4 tsp. Of EVOO.

- Bake at 375 degrees for about 50 minutes or until tender when poked with a fork.

Tomato Potato Soup

Ingredients:
6 cups of filtered water without fluoride
1 pound of fresh mushrooms. Wash and remove stems.)
1 Tablespoon minced garlic
3 medium tomatoes (washed and cored)
1 green pepper (washed, seeded and stem removed)
1 small onion, peeled
1 teaspoon sea salt (See Index: Salt Example)
1 Tablespoon dried parsley

1/4 teaspoon cayenne pepper
1/4 cup EVOO (extra virgin olive oil)
6 medium washed & scrubbed potatoes (about 3 pounds)

What to do:
The night before:
In Crock Pot on low heat:
- Add first three ingredients into crock pot with lid. Cook on low head for 8-to-10 hours.

In the morning in blender:
- Add one at a time and blend after each: tomatoes, green pepper, onion, salt, parsley, cayenne and EVOO.

- Add filtered water without fluoride as necessary to raise mixture level in blender bowl to almost 5.5 cups.

- Add half of mixture to crock pot.

- Pick out mushrooms with a slotted spoon and add to blender.

- Blend.

On a Cutting Board:
- Wash potatoes with scrub brush.

- Cut off bad places off skin and cut into bite-size pieces. Leave unblemished potato skin on potato.

- Add to crock pot and stir well.

- Cook on low heat for 8-to-10 more hours.

Ideas: Tomato/Potato Juice leftover options:
1) Put juice on a baked potato

2) Add leftover veggies and some leftover non-hormone meat.

3) Add new veggies and simmer for 20 minutes until veggies are tender. (Like a mini, one-person soup.)

4) Pour over brown rice.

5) Pour this juice in a fry pan, add a little whole wheat flour and make into a gravy. (About 1 teaspoon per cup of juice.)

Tomato Soup (Creamy)

Ingredients:
1 pound carrots
1 pound white potatoes
1 teaspoon sea salt (See Index: Salt Example)
1/2 teaspoon red pepper seeds (optional)
6-to-8 cloves of garlic (peeled)
1 Recipe Strained tomatoes in this book

What to do: Crock Pot:
- **Boil 10 cups of filtered water without fluorideand add to crock pot.**

- **Cut carrots & white potatoes in quarters.**

- **Add veggies to crock.**

- **Add salt, peeled garlic and optional red pepper seeds.**

- **Cover crock pot with lid on high heat for 8 hours**

- **Veggies are VERY tender.**

- **Take off the lid and allow to cool for at least one hour.**

- **Mash veggies with a potato masher.**

- Use wand mixer and make smooth. Sometimes this is a little difficult not to spray the entire kitchen with sauce, so I transfer the cooled ingredients into a blender and puree the sauce until smooth and put back in the blender.

- Stir in strained tomato recipe.

Don't tell your family or guests what this REALLY is until dinner is done or if someone asks you. No one needs to know this is good for them. Shhhhh – it is a secret.

This recipe is also fantastic when you have a cold or feel one coming. Soup is easier for your body to digest and that means you are giving your body less to digest and more time to put your immune system into action.

Turkey

At least two times a year I have turkey. Why? Because it is easy and I can cook a large turkey (15-to-20 pounds) with the same energy it takes for me to cook a smaller one. I'm not talking about the energy it takes to cook the bird. I'm talking about the energy it takes me to prepare it. So, who saves the energy? I do.

The only trick to this recipe is having a roasting pan large enough that has a good-fitting lid. Never use aluminum foil or those cheap aluminum roasting pans. According to the experts, aluminum is absorbed by the brain and may be linked to Alzheimer's disease. An enamel-coated roaster works well.

Try to get a free-range turkey from your health food store or butcher. Sometimes they will make a special order for an extra large free-range turkey, sometimes not. But, around the holidays, they may stock a "free-range turkey." That's the buzz word for a non-hormone turkey—— "Free range."

If you cannot find one, just do your best. Never get a self-basting turkey. They are pumped with "Poison" you shouldn't eat. Save money and save your health by getting a plain turkey. They are usually cheaper than the self-basting type.

What to do:
- **Remove neck, giblets (inside chest cavity of bird), any plastic that hold the feet together, thermometer or anything foreign from a live, living bird that you might see on a farm. Remove the giblets —usually under the flap of skin where the neck used to be. (I throw this away. Some cooks use as a base for their chicken broth.)**

- **Wash turkey under warm running water.**

- **Give turkey a massage using EVOO or Garlic EVOO all over bird.**

- **Lightly sprinkle sea salt over entire bird.**

- **Put 2 rounded Tablespoons of Minced Garlic inside bird cavity.**

- **Put 1/4 inch of filtered water without fluoride in pan and put the bird in the pan.**

- **Bake at 400 degrees for 1 hour with the lid off.**

- Bake with lid and cook overnight at 150 degrees (about 8-to-10 hours.)

Example:
15 pound bird will cook about 6 hours at 150 degrees with the lid on. (after 1 hour at 400 degrees with the lid off.)

NOTE: When you wake up, the smell is wonderful. When the turkey is cool, meat should fall off the bone. For leftovers: Divide meat and wrap in wax paper. Then put into freezer bags in serving sizes. Freeze for another lazy day.

True Confession from a lazy, sneaky cook – that would be me:

One year I didn't pre-order my organic turkey. Oops. So, I bought an organic chicken - much smaller, and prepared it the exact same way as this recipe suggests. Everyone was surprised at my purchase of a small turkey. Did I open my mouth to tell them it was a small chicken? And break the family tradition of eating turkey every year? NOPE! Sorry. Did my family know? NOPE! Are you gonna tell them? NOPE! Remember, you are sworn to secrecy that the recipes in this book AIN'T healthy it's just good-tasting food.

This secret stuff is more important than you may realize

Veggie Casserole

Ingredients:
1/8-to-1/4 teaspoon cayenne (optional)
1 cup brown rice
1 teaspoon turmeric
2-1/2 cups filtered water without fluoride

1/4 cup EVOO
1 teaspoon homemade minced garlic
4-to-5 cups cleaned, bite-size veggies*
What to do:

- *Get creative with this yummy dish. You can add all your family's favorite veggies. Change the veggies and you have changed the entire personality of the dish. No one will know you are using the same recipe.

- 12 by 9 inch baking pan:

- Add all of the ingredients above.

- Stir together

- Put a stainless steel cookie sheet on top. (this is not work without the cookie sheet on top.)

- Bake 400 degrees for about 90 minutes. All the water will be absorbed.

- Serve with homemade bread and salad. Want meat? Put chicken on the grill and use the left-over chicken for sandwiches instead of using unhealthy lunch meats.

- Creative Options: Pick the veggies you like. Here are a few 4-cup combinations that have worked for me:

- Zucchini (yellow and/or green)

- Peas & corn (frozen works well)

- Bell peppers and green beans

- Bell peppers for all four cups

- Green beans for all four cups

Leftovers:
In the morning, I put the leftovers in an iron skillet for 5 minutes on medium heat—until warm. Then push them over to the side, add some EVOO, and fry a free-range chicken egg for breakfast. Fast and yummy! Two of my favorites cooking words.

Vegetable Soup

Ingredients:
3 cups tomato juice (Ingredients say: tomatoes and salt)
4 cups homemade chicken broth OR filtered water without fluoride
1 Tablespoon Italian Seasoning
1 teaspoon lemon juice or apple cider vinegar
1 Tablespoon chili powder .(check the ingredients on the "chili powder." If the words have any word on it that you don't understand – like flavoring? Find another brand. Organic is an excellent choice for herbs.
4 cups frozen vegetables
1 can of beans, drained & rinsed OR home canned. Ingredients: beans, water salt

What to do:
In 4 quart pot:
- **Add tomato juice, broth, Italian Seasonings, lemon juice and chili powder.**

- **Bring to a boil and then let simmer for 25 minutes.**

- **When tomato mixture changes color, it's ready to add veggies and beans.**

- **Let simmer 10 more minutes.**

- **Serve hot with a slice of toasted whole wheat bread.**

Variation:

If you like chicken vegetable soup, add two cups of shredded chicken breasts before 10-minute simmer time.

Yummy Pockets I

Ingredients:
Flat Bread Recipe
1 teaspoon sea salt (See Index: Salt Example)
3/4 teaspoon ground cumin
1 teaspoon chili powder .(check the ingredients on the "chili powder." If the words have any word on it that you don't understand – like flavoring? Find another brand. Organic is an excellent choice for herbs.
1 medium onion chopped
4 stalks chopped celery
2 cups shredded chicken (One bag of Make-Ahead Shredded Chicken)

What to do:
This is great disguise for leftovers.
Dough:
- **Form dough into golf-sized balls.**

- **Then roll out with a rolling pin into five-inch circles. Use a bowl upside down to cut dough into a circle. (Don't take a lot of time with this. You'll go batty!)**

In Large Bowl:
- **Add salt, cumin and chili powder to a bowl. .(check the ingredients on the "chili powder." If the words have any word on it that you don't understand – like flavoring?**

Find another brand. Organic is an excellent choice for herbs.

- **Mix spices with spoon.**
- **Add onion/celery and meat.**
- **Blend with rubber spatula.**

Variation Note:
If your family likes onion, use one medium onion and four stalks of celery. If they don't like onion, use more celery or all celery. DON'T TELL ANY ONE! Believe me, they won't know.

To stuff into pockets:
- Put 1-1/2-to-2 Tablespoons of the stuffing into each circle. Fold over dough and press edges with a fork. Gently place on a baking sheet with EVOO liberally applied. (No need to let rise.) Bake for 15-to-20 minutes at 350 degrees.
- Yummy Pockets freeze well for eating fast snacks and lunches on the run.
- Bake for 10 or 15 minutes at 350 degrees. Also, good to eat at room temperature for a packed lunch from home.

Yummy Pockets II

Ingredients:
Flat bread
Italian Salmon Recipe (1/2-to-1 pound before cooking)
1 medium onion chopped (varies)
4 stalks chopped celery (varies)

NOTE:
The Italian Salmon can be used by itself without the onion or celery. It's yummy, too.

What to do:
- Same as Yummy Pockets I

- Stuff with wild salmon

Yummy Pockets III

Ingredients:
Mock Sausage
1 medium onion chopped (varies)
4 stalks chopped celery (varies)

What to do:
Same as Yummy Pocket I, but with new stuffing

Idea:
Put a little leftover Simple Crock Spaghetti Sauce on top?
Maybe a little goat's milk cheese on top of the sauce, too?

Baked Beans

Ingredients:
2 cups of white dry navy beans (washed and picked over)
1 Tablespoon minced garlic
6 cups of filtered water without fluoride that is boiling HOT (If the water isn't boiling, this might not work.)
1 cup filtered water without fluoride
1 small onion
1/4 cup unsulphered black strap molasses
3/4 cup raw honey
2 teaspoons dry mustard
1 teaspoon sea salt (See Index: Salt Example)

What to do:
In a crock pot for overnight cooking:
- Add dry beans, garlic and HOT water.

- Cover crock-pot with lid.

- Put on low heat for 8-to-10 hours.

- In the morning, in a blender:

- Add water, onion, molasses, honey, dry mustard and salt.

- Blend. Drain water from crock-pot and rinse beans.

- Return beans to crock-pot.

- Add blender ingredients to the crock-pot.

- Stir into beans.

- Slow cook on low heat for 7-to-8 more hours without the lid.

Baked Potato

This is my favorite food because it is fast and easy. Two words I love to use in the same sentence. Since my duck research, I NEVER eat the skin.

Ingredient:
One Large White Potato (or more. I fill the oven and let cool. Then I put them into a bowl, cover and store in the refrigerator for a fast side dish by frying until golden brown in EVOO in an iron skillet.

What to do:
- **Wash potato with a food scrub brush**

- **Puncture with a knife a few times (prevents the potato from exploding in the oven.)**

- **Place each potato on stainless steel cookie sheet. Never use Teflon for the same reasons why you would never use aluminum. What's that? The Teflon will leech or flake into your food.**

- **Bake potato for 1 hour at 400 degrees. (Time varies.)**

You will know your potato is fully cooked when a fork can slide into the potato and out again very effortlessly.

Bruschetta Gargoyle Bread

When my grandson was three he asked, "Nana, I want some of that gargoyle bread." After much quizzing, I discovered that Jake's gargoyle bread was really "garlic oil bread."

Garlic oil is a healer. Hippocrates said, "Let your food be your medicine, let medicine be your food." When we eat gargoyle bread our food is our medicine. This food makes you feel good. The Italians have a different name for Gargoyle bread, they call it Bruschetta.

Ingredients:
Bread from this cook book
Garlic EVOO
Oregano or Italian Seasonings
Dry Goat's milk grated cheese
Medium tomato
What to do:
- **Paint or dip each slice of bread into Garlic EVOO.**

- Sprinkle on some oregano or Italian
- Seasonings.
- Wash, core and dice a tomato.
- Place a liberal amount of tomato on each slice of bread.
- Sprinkle on some cheese.
- Put on a 13 X 9 baking dish or cookie sheet.
- Bake 10-to-15 minutes at 350 degrees. (bread should be lightly toasted and cheese melted.)

Candied Carrots

Ingredients:
2 pounds carrots
1 cup filtered water without fluoride
1/4 cup raw honey
1/4 cup EVOO

What to do:
- **Wash and scrape carrots clean**
- **Cut into bite-size pieces**
- **Place in a glass or stainless steel baking dish**
- **Combine EVOO (extra Virgin Olive Oil) and honey and stir to combine**
- **Drizzle over carrots**

- Put on lid or place a cookie sheet over the dish.

- Bake for one hour at 350 degree.

- Puncture with a fork to make sure they are very tender. If not, cook for five-to-10 more minutes.

Candied Yams

Ingredients:
One Sweet Potato
Raw honey
3 or 4 Tablespoons EVOO (extra virgin olive oil)
Ground cinnamon for sprinkle

What to do:
- Bake sweet potato (Yam)

- Let cool.

- Cut in Half.

- Slather 1 teaspoon of EVOO on baking dish

- Place sweet potato on the baking dish

- Drizzle on one Tablespoon of raw honey on each half of potato.

- Paint EVOO on each potato or slather using your fingers.

- Lightly Sprinkle ground cinnamon on top (optional)

- Bake in a glass pan at 350 degrees for about 10 min.

If you need a larger serving, just multiply. Allow one sweet potato per person, and one extra for the baking dish.

Chicken Soup (Creamy)

Ingredients:
3 quarts homemade chicken broth from this book
6 cloves of garlic
Peeled (about one ounce.)
3 pounds potatoes
1 teaspoon sea salt (See Index: Salt Example)

<u>**What to do:**</u>
In the Crock pot:

- **Add all ingredients.**

- **Put on the lid. Cook on low heat for 10 hours.**

- **Let cool (two or three hours)**

- **Puree all ingredients. I have a wand blender and it makes this task much easier than a food processor or a regular blender. I can blend right in the crock pot.**

NOTE:

This creamy broth can be used as a standalone soup or as a base to a chicken soup -- without or without meat. Put in your favorite veggies cut into bite-size pieces. Return to the crock pot on medium heat for an additional 8 more hours.

Broth substitute: If you don't have three quarts of chicken broth sitting in the freezer, you can remove the skin of some organic chicken. Put it in a pot and boil it with a full pot of filtered water without fluoride. (usually 10-to-16 cups) By the way, a quart is equal to four cups of water. Add 1 Tablespoon minced garlic and 1 teaspoon sea salt. Boil until the chicken is white and flaky.

Store-bought chicken broth is mostly chemicals and the chicken walks through the broth wearing stilts.

Chicken Salad Sandwiches

Ingredients:
One package of homemade shredded chicken from freezer—thawed. OR boil your non-hormone, free range chicken in filtered water without fluoride and 1 teaspoon minced garlic..
4 stalks of celery
1 small onion (optional)

What to do:
In medium bowl:

- **Add chopped celery and onion mixture (to your family's preference—about one cup)**

- **Mix meat (about two cups cooked) and celery mixture with one of the following options.**

Variation 1: EVOO Salad Dressing (Fold in with rubber spatula)

Variation 2: EVOO Mustard (Fold in with rubber spatula)

Variation 3: EVOO or Garlic EVOO brushed or lightly spread onto bread. Then lightly sprinkle with oregano. Add mixture onto bread.

Serve on whole wheat bread, and with soup.

Store-bought bread?

Ezekiel 4:9 bread **used to be okay** bread. Sad to say, but Food Manufacturers change their methods of manufacturing when they can cut a corner to increase their profits. Good for them but bad for consumers.

Two things wrong:
1) they now add malted barley flour. The process of malting is a way to ferment the barley. That should be beneficial to consumers, but most Food Manufacturers use chemicals to ferment the food quickly. The chemicals are the danger.

2) This bread company adds "gluten" to their bread. That is not natural. Gluten is part of the wheat flour. Adding extra gluten means that flour somewhere was stripped of its gluten to make this bread. Extra gluten makes this bread UN-natural and I no longer have a store-bought bread to recommend. Bummer.

Let the buyer beware!!

Each time I grocery shop it is an adventure to see how "THEY" want to "TRICK" me. I always watched a program on television with Angela Lansbury called, "Murder She Wrote." I liked the twists and turns of the plot. I could NEVER guess how any of the programs would end.

I have tried my best to take this "fun" attitude with me into the grocery store, and think of the games that Food Manufacturers are playing are a game of me against "them." If I didn't have this attitude, I believe that grocery shopping would be too frustrating.

Corn and Potato Casserole

Ingredients:
2-1/2 pounds potatoes
1/2 cup EVOO
1 Tablespoon raw honey
1 large onion
1 pound frozen corn
1 Tablespoon dried parsley
1/2 Tablespoon sea salt (See Index: Salt Example)
1 cup filtered water without fluoride
1/4 cup whole wheat flour
Paprika to sprinkle on top

What to do:

If someone in your family does not like corn, then this is a sneaky way to get your children to eat their veggies because your blender purees the corn so everyone thinks the corn is just a yummy sauce.

- **Peel and slice potatoes thin. I use a food processor.**
- **Distribute potatoes nicely in a 12" by 9" baking dish**

In Blender:
- **Add EVOO, honey, onion (quartered)**
- **Puree.**
- **Add frozen corn, parsley, salt and water**

- Puree

- Strain any corn pieces out. If your family doesn't mind corn, you can skip this step.

- Add whole-wheat flour

- Puree

- Pour blender ingredients over potatoes

- Poke potatoes down into sauce so they are almost completely covered.

- Lightly sprinkle paprika on top.

- Bake from cold over at 350 for one hour and ten minutes.

- Potatoes are very tender when you poke them with a fork.

Please note:
This is MY comfort food. Mom made this and I LOVED it. Of course, it was canned cream style corn—deadly—but this is pretty close to the taste, but food as medicine. Great memories sitting around the table as a child with my family.

Corn Bread Stuffing

Ingredients:
1 whole garlic head (peeled)
1 whole bell pepper (cored and washed)
1 pound onions (peeled)
4-to-5 stalks celery (washed, leaves off)
1 pound carrots (washed & skin lightly scraped.)
1 cup home-made chicken broth

1 can homemade beans (pinto or white) or store bought beans and delete salt.
1/4-to-1/8 teaspoon ground cayenne pepper
1 teaspoon sea salt (See Index: Salt Example)
1 corn bread recipe in this book
3/4 cup chopped pecans (optional)

What to do:
Note: I use a food processor for slicing veggies:
- **Slice garlic, pepper, onion, celery.**

- **Grate carrots. This equals about 11 cups.**

Iron Skillet:
- Add a 1/2 cup EVOO

- Add food processor veggies

- Cook on medium heat with the lid off. 20-to-30 minutes

- Veggies are soft.

Blender:
- **Add homemade chicken broth**

- **Add beans**

- **Add salt (eliminate if you use store-bought canned beans with salt added.**

- **Cayenne (I use 1/4 teaspoon)**

- **Blend until smooth**

Large Bowl:
- **Crumble entire baked corn bread recipe into the bowl.**

- **Add skillet and blender ingredients.**

- Mix well

- 1 teaspoon of EVOO in 12 by 9 glass pan, and spread with your fingers

- Pour into baking pan evenly

- Sprinkle nuts on top

- Bake at 350 degrees for 1 hour.

Egg Salad

Ingredients:
4 organic chicken eggs hard boiled
EVOO Salad Dressing
1 stalk celery chopped
1/2 small onion, chopped

What to do:
In a Pot:
- Boil eggs at a rolling boil for 10 minutes

- Cool, Peel and Chop

- Add EVOO Salad Dressing to cover all the eggs.

- Add one stalk of chopped celery

- Add 1/2 chopped onion (optional)

- Stir in dressing. Put as little or as much as you like of the dressing—it's good for you.

Serving Ideas:
- Serve on organic bread

- Wrap in a lettuce leaf like a taco.

Macaroni Salad

Ingredients:
2 cups dry whole wheat noodles
1 small onion diced (optional)
4 hard-boiled, free-range chicken eggs
1 cup thawed frozen peas
2 small, whole tomatoes, washed, cored and diced
1 teaspoon sea salt (See Index: Salt Example)
1/4 teaspoon black pepper (optional)
6 stalks small diced celery
1/2-to-3/4 cup EVOO mustard
What to do:
In a 4-quart pot:
- **Cook noodles until done. (Whole wheat noodles need to be cooked a longer than enriched noodles.)**

- **Drain noodles.**

In a mixing bowl:
- **Add the remaining ingredients**

- **Stir in "EVOO Mustard." Use enough mustard so every noodle is coated or to your family's preference.**

Mashed Potatoes

Ingredients:
Mixing Bowl full of peeled and washed raw potatoes (About three pounds.)
3 Tablespoons of EVOO
(Garlic EVOO makes garlic mashed potatoes)
1 Tablespoon minced garlic

1 teaspoon sea salt (See Index: Salt Example)
1 cup-to-1-1/2 cups filtered water without fluoride
1 teaspoon raw honey

What to do:
- Boil potatoes in filtered water without fluoride until done.

- Drain water.

- Put in mixing bowl.

- Add EVOO.

- Add minced garlic.

- Add sea salt.

- Add filtered water without fluoride and honey.

- Slowly add water and honey to bowl and mix with a hand mixer. Beat until fluffy or your family's preference.

Okra and Tomatoes

Ingredients:
2 large tomatoes (washed and cored)
1 red or yellow onion, peeled
1 Tablespoon minced garlic
1 teaspoon sea salt (See Index: Salt Example)
1 Tablespoon Italian Seasoning
1/8-to-1/4 teaspoon cayenne pepper
1 pound fresh or frozen okra cut into
bite-size pieces with stems removed

What to do:
In blender:
- **Add tomatoes, (one at a time) onion in quarters, garlic, salt, Italian seasoning and cayenne.**

In large pot:
- **Add blender mixture**

- **Add frozen or fresh okra**

- **Stir together until okra is coated with mixture.**

- **Cook on low heat until okra is tender.**

Perfect Brown Rice

Ingredients:
2 cups of brown rice (not from a box)
4 cups of filtered water without fluoride OR homemade chicken broth

What to do:
In a 12 x 9-inch glass baking dish:
- Add rice and water to baking dish.

- Bake in the oven with a cookie sheet on top at 350 degrees for 1-hour to 1-hour, 10 minutes. This will NOT work without the cookie sheet on top to keep the steam in. Please do NOT use aluminum foil.

Optional:
One stalk celery - wash and slice small—it's a little bit of color and flavor. (You will know the rice is done when you cannot see bubbles in the baking dish.)

NOTE:
If you don't put the stainless steel cookie sheet on top, this won't work! Never use aluminum or aluminum foil. You can use an enamel cookie sheet if you cannot find stainless steel. Go to my website to see the kitchen ware I suggest.

Stuffed Mushrooms

Ingredients:
1 can wild salmon (6 ounce can) drained
1 cup Homemade bread crumbs
1/4 cup garlic oil OR 1/4 cup EVOO with one teaspoon of minced garlic mixed together
1 small onion, chopped or stalk of celery
1 pound mushrooms (cleaned and stems removed.)

Topping:
Lightly sprinkle Paprika and Goat's milk cheese

What to do:
In a bowl:
- **Mix salmon, (liquid drained and rinsed) breadcrumbs, garlic oil, and onion or celery.**

- **Stuff mixture into clean mushrooms.**

- **Put in a glass baking dish that has been slathered with your fingers with EVOO.**

- **Lightly sprinkle with goats milk cheese and paprika (optional for color)**

- **Bake for 40 minutes at 350 degrees.**

Tabouleh (Pronounced - Tah-BOO-lee)

Ingredients:
1-1/2 cups whole wheat bulgur
(7-to-8 ounces)
3 cups boiling filtered water without fluoride
1 cup minced fresh parsley
1 medium tomato, finely chopped (washed and cored)
1/2 cup chopped green onions
(use the green part, too)
2 Tablespoons minced or chopped fresh mint leaves
1/2 cup chopped pecans (optional)
1/4 cup lemon juice
1 teaspoon sea salt (See Index: Salt Example)
1 pinch-to-1/8 teaspoon of cayenne pepper
2 Tablespoons EVOO

What to do:
In four-cup measuring cup or bowl:
- Stir together bulgur and water.

- Let soak for one hour. Most of water will be absorbed.

In large mixing bowl:
- **Add parsley, tomato, green onions, mint leaves and optional pecans.**

- **Squeeze out excess moisture from bulgur.**

- **Add bulgur to large mixing bowl.**

- **Salad Dressing in small bowl:**

- **Whisk together lemon juice, sea salt, cayenne and EVOO.**

- Pour dressing over large mixing bowl of salad ingredients.

- Toss to combine.

- Cover and refrigerate until chilled before serving.

Corn Bread

Ingredients:
1-cup whole wheat flour
3/4 cup un-enriched cornmeal
1 teaspoon baking soda
1 cup filtered water without fluoride
2 Tablespoons EVOO
2 Tablespoons unsulphered black- strap molasses
1 free-range chicken egg (optional)

What to do:
In mixing bowl:
- Add whole wheat flour.

- Mix, cornmeal and baking soda together with a fork. Crush any lumps.

- Add to mixing bowl.

- In 2-cup mixing cup:

- Mix: water, EVOO, molasses & egg.

- Beat with fork for about 30 seconds.

- Add to mixing bowl and fold in with a rubber spatula. (Looks like cake batter.)

- **Spread 1 Tablespoon of EVOO with fingers or brush with a basting brush on pan.**

- **Bake for 20 minutes at 350 degrees. (Poke with a toothpick to see if done. Toothpick will come out clean)**

Flatbread Easiest Bread to make

This is my favorite bread because I'm LAZY! Sometimes called, "Unleavened Bread" or Flat bread. You can stuff this bread with the egg salad in this book or it is perfect to stuff with leftovers. Put some of your homemade EVOO salad dressing and this is delicious with most any food inside the bread. You can eat this bread plain as a good grab and go snack. No yeast, just flour and water. Ya cannot mess this up. I just use flour and water. I love it. I make a batch or two and have two fry pans going at the same time.

YES, you can freeze this recipe. I put a piece of wax paper between the flatbreads so they do NOT freeze. Then I take the pile of flatbread and the wax paper and put them into a gallon freezer bag. Wonderful. This is truly a magician in the kitchen miracle.

Ingredients:
2 cups whole wheat flour
1-1/4 cups filtered water without fluoride
3 Tablespoons EVOO (extra virgin olive oil)
1 teaspoon sea salt (See Index: Salt Example)
Later:

2 or more additional cups of whole wheat flour

What to do:
In a Large mixing bowl:
- **Add two cups of whole wheat flour and salt**

In a glass measuring cup:
- **Stir measuring cup ingredients into dry ingredients with a spoon or spatula**

Note:

If you want this to become a friendly germ recipe (probiotic) then let the recipe rest at this point overnight. According to Jewish law, fermentation starts after 17 minutes. I like to make this recipe in two sections because it is easier for me to find a small block of time - say 20 minutes - and then another 20 minutes in the morning while I am waiting for breakfast to cook that I start rolling out the dough.

- **Later or continue the recipe without allowing the flour and other ingredients to ferment:**

- **Add a half cup of flour at a time and stir into dough.**

- **Usually one more cup total.**

- **When the dough is too difficult to stir with the spatula, add one cup of flour on the counter top & put the dough on the flour.**

- **No need to knead for a long time—- just keep folding the dough into the dry flour until it gets less sticky and smooth.**

- **Make golf-size balls. (about 12 to 14)**

- **Roll out each ball with a rolling pin to make round flatbread. If you don't have a rolling pin, you can flatten the balls of dough with your finger tips like making pizza dough. About a 1/4 inch thick works well. You can also roll out the dough by using a quart canning jar on its side like you would a rolling pin. Primitive, but it works fine.**

- **Use remainder of the flour to roll out dough for each flatbread. Some flour may be left over - just toss it.**

Last step:
- **Iron skillet on Medium Low Heat:**

- **Place one rolled out flatbread in pre-heated iron skillet. (no EVOO, no nothing—a dry pan)**

- **Cook for about 3 minutes on first side.**

- **Flip and cook the second side for about 1 minute.**

Cooked flatbread may be frozen with wax paper in between each flatbread and then store in a gallon freezer bag. Thaws in under five minutes.

You don't need to cook the whole batch of dough at the same time. Place dough in a glass bowl and cover with saran wrap. Stays in the frig for about a week or week and a half. Roll out as needed.

Flatbread is a wonderful way to eat leftovers or as my grandmother used to call it "Ice Box Special."

Organic Bread

A great yeast-free bread with friendly germs to help anyone with stomach problems, constipation or IBS disease. This recipe tastes too sour for me to eat every day. I prefer the Lazy Bread recipe in this book for every day eating. You be the judge.

Three Steps:

Step One: Making the Starter

Another descriptive word for this might be: "Making Home Made Yeast." Starter has no other word that I can relate to here in the 21st century. A meaningless word to me? Baking bread this way is actually easier than using store-bought yeast. With store bought yeast you must make warm water for the yeast. If the water is too cold, the yeast won't be activated. If the water is too hot, you will kill the yeast. This method doesn't require making warm water to activate the yeast.

Ingredients:
2 cups of whole-wheat flour
2 cups of filtered water without fluoride.

What to do:
In a Blender: (or in a bowl is fine if you don't have a blender)

- **Add flour and water**

- **Blend or stir together.**

- **Scrape sides.**

- **Blend until smooth and creamy or stir.**

- In a very large glass mixing bowl:

- Add Blender ingredients to the bowl. Use a rubber spatula to scrape blender sides.

- Put a cotton dish towel on top (keep out of drafts)

- Let stand two days (no need to stir in-between.)

- Don't put bowl in a cabinet. The good germs need to stop by on the counter top.

- Wait 24 hours.

Please Note: If contamination occurs, you will need to scald the bowl with hot water and start over. Contamination will have a disagreeable color like orange or blue PLUS have a disagreeable odor. Please see "Fermenting Basics

Organic Bread Step Two

Okay your yeast (Starter) has been sitting on the counter for 48 hours. NEXT!

Ingredients: (second time)
2 cups of whole-wheat flour
2 cups of filtered water without fluoride.

What to do:
In a Blender: (or in a bowl is fine if you don't have a blender)
- Add flour and water

- Blend or stir.

- Scrape sides once.

- Blend or stir until smooth and creamy

- Add this to the starter you made yesterday and let stand another 8 hours:

- Stir Blender ingredients and the yeast or starter together.

- Once combined, remove one cup of mixture into a glass measuring cup. This is your home made yeast or "starter" for your next organic bread.

- Cover and store in the refrigerator.

- Now you have roughly three cups of mixture left in the bowl: You are ready to make your first loaf of bread.

Organic Bread Step Three or

Your first loaf of Organic Bread

Ingredients:
2 cups of whole wheat flour
1/2 cup raw honey
1/2 cups EVOO
Later: 4 more cups will be used - see the instructions below.
What to do:

- Stir the above flour, honey and EVOO into the three cups of flour and water with your spatula

- Add one cup whole wheat flour and stir into flour

- Add one more cup of flour and stir into flour

- Use your hands when too difficult to stir with the spatula

- Put one cup of flour on the counter

- Put dough on top of flour.

- Put one more cup flour on top of the dough and knead.

- Knead means putting the dry flour on top of the dough and folding it into the flour.

- You will NOT use all of the last two cups of flour - - depending how energetic you are, how much patience you have, and your baking experience. Don't sweat it, just put that dough together so it is not too sticky. A little sticky is okay.

In two-one pound glass loaf pans:
- Add one Tablespoon of EVOO in each pan and slather on bottom and sides of pan. (Slather means—use your fingers to spread the oil around.)

- Divide dough equally. Knead and then put into two loaf pans and pat down.

- Use a knife to make a light scoring on the top of each bread - length wise.

- I put pans in my cold oven for 4-to-12 hours, uncovered to rise.

- Bread should rise by 1/4 to 1/2 size larger.

- Bake at 350 degrees from a cold oven about 45 minutes.

- Let bake until golden brown. (keep checking every 10 minutes or so.).

- Let cool about 30 minutes.

- Use a knife to cut around all four sides to separate bread from pan.

- When cool, bread should fall out.

- Slice and eat.

This bread is wonderful for freezing. I slice each loaf with my electric slicing machine, wrap 3 or 4 slices of bread in wax paper and then put into freezer bags. Thaws in a few minutes, or you can toast frozen bread.

This is truly food as medicine. Congrats from one NUT to another.

Organic Bread, Second Loaf

Ingredients:
2 cups of whole-wheat flour
2 cups of filtered water without fluoride
1 cup starter

What to do:
- Put flour water and starter into your blender
- Blend until smooth.

- Scrape sides and blend again.

- Pour into a large bowl

- Cover with a cotton dishtowel and let sit on the counter top for 8-to 24 hours.

- After waiting Stir well together.

- Remove one cup of the mixture to put into a glass container in the refrigerator this is your new Starter)

- In a measuring cup:

- 1/2 cup of raw honey

- 1/2 cup of EVOO

- Stir measuring cup ingredients into flour and water.

- Add one more cup of whole-wheat flour

- Stir well.

- Add another cup of whole-wheat flour

- Stir well.

- At this point it may be too difficult to combine.

- Put one more cup of flour on the counter top.

- Scrape out the dough mixture onto the flour on the counter top.

- Add one more cup of flour on top of dough to begin kneading. (Keep folding the dough into the dry flour. When flour is smooth and not too sticky, you are ready to let it rise.

In two-one pound glass loaf pans: (stainless steel is fine, too)

- Add one Tablespoon of EVOO in each pan and slather on bottom and sides of pan. (Slather means—use your fingers.)

- Divide dough equally. Knead and then press into two loaf pans and pat down.

- Use a knife to make a light scoring on the top of each bread - length wise.

- I put pans in my cold oven for 4-to-12 hours, uncovered to rise.

- Bread should rise by 1/4 to 1/2 size larger.

- Bake at 350 degrees from a cold oven about 45 minutes. Let bake until golden brown. (keep checking every 10 minutes.)

- Let cool about 30 minutes.

- Use a knife to cut around all four sides to separate bread from pan.

- Once cooled, the bread should pop out with the help of a fork when you turn it upside-down.

- Slice and eat.

Pizza Crust (Thin)

The longer I eat this diet, the lazier I become. Imagine that? Here's my version of crunchy pizza crust:

Ingredients:
Flatbread from the recipe in this book. I can take the flatbread I need right out of my freezer.
Spaghetti Sauce in this book or puree some washed, raw tomatoes
Black olives (Ingredients: ripe olives, water and sea salt – nothing else)

Sautee chopped onions (optional)
Goat's milk cheese

What to do:
In an iron skillet on medium heat:

- **¼ cup EVOO**

- **Once the oil is warm, I place my flatbread in the oil and brown one side.**

- **Flip the flatbread**

- **Add chopped black olives and optional chopped and cooked onions**

- **Add sauce**

- **Sprinkle goat's milk cheese the way you like it.**

- **Cover the pan with a lid and remove from heat.**

- **Let rest for about 3-to-5 minutes. (The cheese is melted.)**

Makes one serving. You can have two fry pans going to save time, and let each person put what they like on their pizza

Bread or Irish Soda Bread

Ingredients:
4 cups of whole wheat flour
1 teaspoon baking soda
2 teaspoons apple cider vinegar
1 teaspoon blackstrap molasses (Ingredients MUST say, "unsulphered")
1-3/4 cups filtered water without fluoride

What to do:
A Yummy Bread for when you don't have time or inclination to wait for the dough to rise. That would be me.

In very large mixing bowl:
- Add 2 cups of flour

- Add baking soda stir with fork or whisk.

In a two-cup measuring cup:
- Add water, molasses, apple cider vinegar and extra virgin olive oil (EVOO)

- Add this measuring cup to the dry ingredients.

- Start mixing with a large spoon to combine.

- Add one cup more of flour.

- When too difficult, use your hands.

- Add more flour until dough is stiff. Do not over mix the flour. You are combining the ingredients, and then stop.

- Place ball into a one-pound, glass loaf dish that has had about 1 Tablespoon of EVOO smeared on it. (Use your fingers for smearing.)

- Push dough down into the pan to make dough flat into the dish, and then pick up the dough and flip it so the dough has EVOO on it. (I'm soooo lazy!)

- Use a knife to lightly score the top of the dough.

- Bake at 350 degrees from a cold oven for about 40-to-45 minutes. (Bread should be lightly brown on the top, and toothpick comes out clean from the thickest part of the bread.)

- Hand slice at the table or use a bread slicer for thin slices.)

- Serve plain, or add peanut butter, or mock mayonnaise, or apple butter or raw honey.

- I love to dip this bread into the EVOO Salad Dressing from this book.

Note:
I make bread sticks with this dough, too. Make golf-sized balls and roll out into sticks. I sometimes lightly sprinkle each bread stick with canning. Bake at 350 degrees for about 20 minutes.

Freezing:
I slice the bread with my bread slicer and then wrap three or four pieces in wax paper. I place the bundles into a gallon freezer bag & freeze. When you need some bread, take out a bundle and before the sandwich is made, the bread is thawed. Toasting the bread makes it taste sweeter and makes the bread faster to eat.

Chocolate Cake

Ingredients:
2 teaspoons baking soda
2 cups whole wheat flour OR whole wheat pastry flour

1 can crushed pineapple in its own juice (20 ounce size) OR 2 cups of blended fresh pineapple
1/4 cup EVOO
3/4 cup raw honey
6 Tablespoons Baker's Cocoa (Ingredients say: Chocolate (that's it. Double this amount for Chocolate lovers.)
2 Tablespoons EVOO
Topping Options:
1 cup chopped nuts (I like pecans) OR Frosting from this cookbook.

NOTE:
If you don't make the frosting, I use chopped nuts for the topping. Add chopped nuts to the top of batter before baking.

What to do:
In a large mixing bowl:
- **Add baking soda, cocoa and whole wheat flour.**
- **Stir with a fork, mashing any lumps in**
- **baking soda or cocoa.**

In a blender:
- **Add pineapple with juice, EVOO, Honey, and EVOO**
- **In a large mixing bowl:**
- **Add blender ingredients to dry flour**
- **mixture. Use a rubber spatula to scrape blender bowl into mixing bowl.**
- **Fold into flour with spatula.**

Layer Cake:
- **Divide evenly between two cake pans sprayed with EVOO.**

- **Bake at 350 for 30-to 35 minutes. Toothpick will come out clean.**

NOTE:
Frosting is spread in the middle of the cake between the two layers, and for the top. Sprinkle one cup of nuts on frosting.

LAZY Sheet-Cake Method (No Frosting)

What to do:
- **Pour the entire batter into a 13 by 9 pan that has EVOO sprayed on it.**

- **Sprinkle one cup of nuts on top.**

- **Lightly pat in.**

- **Bake at 350 for 35-to-45 minutes (toothpick comes out clean)**

NOTE:
Most cake is too sweet for me. I find myself shaving off the frosting with my fork. This cake just right. You might not like it——too plain. The frosting adds extra sweetness to this cake. Remember: Sweet is an "acquired" taste. The less you eat, the less you want. Experiment.

According to Dr. David Reuben, it is cheaper for a Food Manufacturer to put sugar in your store-bought cake mix than it is to put flour. Consequently, the first ingredient to "scratch" cake mixes is sugar! It's no surprise that sugar makes you fat, but did you know that sugar slows down your immune system? Next time you get a cold, take a sugar inventory of your diet.

Sugar also causes an imbalance in your body. Food processing causes sugar to be nutrient free and without the balance that raw, honey naturally has. An unbalanced food causes an unbalanced person—emotionally and physically! Unbalanced food causes "cravings."

Cookies - Graham

Ingredients:
2 cups whole wheat flour
2 teaspoons baking soda
1/2 teaspoon ground cinnamon
1/4 teaspoon nutmeg
1/4 cup EVOO
1/4 cup raw honey
2 Tablespoons blackstrap molasses

What to do:
In large bowl:
- **Add flour, baking soda, cinnamon & nutmeg.**

- **Stir together.**

In a measuring cup:
- **Add EVOO (extra virgin olive oil) honey, molasses**

- **Use hands to make into a dough.**

- **Roll out dough to 1/8" thick**

- **Cut out with cookie cutter or use a round glass.**

- Place on stainless steel cookie sheet.

- Lightly poke cookies with fork all over.

- Bake at 300 degrees in pre-heated oven for 20 min.

- Cool on rack.

Fruit Dessert Layered

Ingredients:
Fancy see-through dessert bowl or goblets
Plain Organic Yogurt (You may need to double the recipe in this book)
Strawberries, chopped
Pineapple chunks
Cookies (from this book)
Use your favorite fruit or fruit that is in season to save some money

What to do:

There aren't any amounts because I don't know how tall your fancy dessert bowl is. This can also be made in fancy goblets as individual servings.

Yes, you can make this recipe the night before your guests arrive. Store in the frig.

How to Layer Ingredients:
- **Cookies (any in this cook book)**
- **Strawberries**
- **Plain yogurt (organic)**

- Pineapples

- Cookies

NOTE:
Top, middle and bottom layers are crumbled cookies.

Cookies - Oatmeal Raisin

Ingredients:
1 free-range chicken egg
1/2 cup EVOO (extra virgin olive oil)
1/2 cup raw honey
1-1/2 cups old fashioned oatmeal
1 teaspoons baking soda
1-1/2 cups whole wheat flour
1 cup raisins

What to do:
Use a hand mixer after adding each ingredient or use a food processor for continuous mixing.

Large Bowl
- **Free-range chicken egg**

- **EVOO (extra virgin olive oil.)**

- **Raw Honey**

- **Whole Wheat Flour**

- **Baking soda**

- **Oats**

- **Raisins**

- Mixture should look like cookie dough.

- Use a Tablespoon to dollop onto stainless steel cookie sheet

- For chewy, bake at 350 degrees for 8 minutes. (slightly brown on top)

- For crunchy, flatten with fork and bake at 350 for about 10 minutes

OPTIONAL:
I like one whole pecan on top of each cookie.

Cookies - Nut Raisin

Ingredients:
1 free-range chicken egg
1/2 cup EVOO (extra virgin olive oil)
3/4 cup raw honey
2 teaspoons baking soda
2 cups whole wheat flour
1 cup raisins
1/2 cup pecans

What to do:
Large Bowl
- Mix Dry Ingredients first:

- Whole Wheat Flour, baking soda, raisins and pecans. Nuts are optional.

- I use my hands to separate the raisins in the flour to make sure that they are not clumped together

- 2-cup glass measuring cup:

- EVOO (extra virgin olive oil.), honey, and egg.

- Blend well with fork

- Add to dry mixture.

- Use spatula to blend and then use your hands.

- Mixture should be fairly stiff.

- If mixtures do not look like cookie dough, add 1/4 cup more flour.

- Use a Tablespoon to dollop onto stainless steel cookie sheet

- Bake at 350 degrees for 8 minutes for chewy

- For crunchy flatten with a fork and bake for 10 minutes

OPTIONAL:
I like one whole pecan on top of each cookie.

Pie Crust Nutty (1 of 3)

Ingredients:
1-1/2 cups of pecans (chopped)
7 Tablespoons of EVOO
2 Tablespoons honey

What to do:
- **Glass Pie Dish: (Stainless steel is fine, too.)**

- **Sprinkle nuts on bottom of pie dish.**

- **Drizzle EVOO on top of nuts.**

- Drizzle honey on top.

- Bake in oven at 350 degrees for about 10-to-5 minutes. Crust is lightly brown.

- Allow to cool. Sometimes I put the crust in the refrigerator to cool quicker.

Pie Crust Two: (2 of 3

Ingredients:
1 cup cookie crumbs (any of the cookies in this book)
1 cup chopped pecans
1/4 cup raw honey
1/2 cup EVOO

What to do:
- Sprinkle cookie crumbs (I like the graham crackers in this recipe book the best.)

- Sprinkle nuts

- In measuring cup:

- Combine raw honey and EVOO (extra virgin olive oil)

- Stir well

- Drizzle on pie pan mixture

- Bake at 350 degrees from cold oven for 10 minutes.

- Let pie crust cool for 20 minutes before you bake in it.

WARNING:

If your home-made pie crust calls for vegetable oil or Crisco, it is deadly for your health. Vegetable oil and Crisco are alternative names for trans fatty acids. Food Manufacturers will sometimes rename their ingredients when they know savvy consumers know that they are unhealthy.

The hint would be an ingredient name you don't know or in this case "vegetable" oil with an un-named vegetable. The FDA allows Food Manufacturers to be vague on their ingredient labels. The front of the label is the "adver-teasing," but the "ingredient list." is your contract. Read your contract!

Pie Crust - Rolled Oats (3 of 3)

Ingredients:
1 cup old fashioned oatmeal (not instant, and not in a pouch)
1/4 cup whole wheat flour
4 Tablespoons EVOO
3 Tablespoons raw honey

What to do:
Preheat oven to 350 degrees:
In a small bowl:

- **Blend oatmeal, flour, EVOO & raw honey.**

- **Fold in with a rubber spatula.**

- **Press into 9-inch pie pan.**

- **Bake at 350 degrees for 10-to-12 minutes.**

Cookies Peanut Butter

My absolute favorite cookie on the planet.

Ingredients:
1/2 cup EVOO (extra virgin olive oil)
1/2 cup raw honey
1/2 cup peanut butter
2 cups whole wheat flour
2 teaspoons baking soda
1/2 cup chopped nuts
Topping: 1 whole pecan on each cookie (optional)

What to do:
2-cup Measuring Cup:
- **Add EVOO (extra virgin olive oil.)**

- **Raw honey.**

- **Peanut butter (ingredients say: peanuts or Peanuts & salt -- that's it!!) or make your own peanut butter from scratch.**

- **Add peanut butter while you watch the measuring cup ingredients rise to 1.5.**

- **Stir until smooth.**

Large Bowl:
- **Add Whole Wheat Flour**

- **Baking soda**

- **Stir baking soda into flour with fork to smash any lumps.**

- **Add measuring cup ingredients. Use spatula to scrape the measuring cup.**

- **Stir all ingredients together with spatula**

- **Finish mixing with hands. (Ahhhhh, more tactile cooking for us mud-pie babies!)**

- **Form into balls (about 1/2 the size of a golf ball)**

- **Put onto a stainless steel baking sheet. (aluminum is NOT good, nor Teflon - both outgas chemicals that gets absorbed into your food. If you cannot find stainless steel, put some parchment paper down on the sheet or use a glass lasagna pan.)**

- **Flatten with a fork.**

- **Put one whole pecan on each cookie (optional)**

- **Bake at 350 degrees for 6-to-8 minutes from a cold oven. 5 minutes in a pre-heated oven.**

- **Second batch takes less time. (6 minutes)**

- **Put cookies on rack to cool.**

WARNING: These cookies go up in smoke FAST! Put on a timer and stay CLOSE! The second reason Food Manufacturers use margarine or Crisco, the smoking point in much higher. The first reason -- it is CHEAPER than EVOO.

Variation: Add some raisins on top or into the cookie dough. This dough freezes well.

Cookies - Protein

Do you have a picky eater? This is a great snack.

Ingredients:
1 cup whole wheat flour
1-1/2 cup Pecan meal
1-1/2 teaspoon baking soda
1 Tablespoon anise
1/2 cup EVOO
1/2 cup raw honey

What to do:
Combine dry ingredients in large mixing bowl:
- **Flour, pecan meal, baking soda & anise.**
- **In a measuring cup combine:**
- **EVOO (extra virgin olive oil) & raw honey**
- **Add measuring cup to large mixing bowl**
- **Mix together to form dough.**
- **Make into half golf ball size.**
- **Press down with a fork on cookie sheet.**
- **Bake for 8 minutes in preheated oven.**
- **Let cool on a cookie rack.**

Optional:
- 1/4 cup of raisins or your favorite nuts.

BEWARE:

Protein shakes have many artificial ingredients in them and cause a long list of health problems -- including joint problems. Eat these cookies instead or have a nice fruit smoothie.

Dessert - Spinach Pie

Ingredients:
2 or 3 carrots
2 medium onions
1 Tablespoon minced garlic
1/2 cup EVOO
2 free-range chicken eggs
8 ounce feta cheese from Goat's milk (if the Feta says, "traditional" don't believe it. Please read the ingredient list.)
1 teaspoon dry mustard powder
1 teaspoon dry dill
2 - 10 ounce packages of frozen spinach -Or- 1 pound fresh spinach

What to do:
Measuring Cup:
- **Grate carrots and onions -- should be three cups.**
- **Defrost spinach and squeeze water out.**

Iron Skillet:
- **1/2 cup EVOO (extra virgin olive oil)**
- **Add measuring cup ingredients**
- **Add minced garlic**
- **Add fresh or frozen spinach**
- **Fry on medium heat with lid on for 20 minutes. Veggies will be tender.**

In Blender:
- 2 free-range chicken eggs

- Add Feta cheese (discard water)

- Add dry mustard and dill

- Puree

Iron Skillet:
- Add Blender ingredients to Fry pan.

- Stir in well and let warm. (about 3-to-5 minutes.)

- 9 inch pie pan:

- 1 Tablespoon EVOO to coat pie pan. (I use my fingers)

- Add Skillet ingredients to pie pan. (do not over fill)

- Bake at 350 degrees for 45 minutes -- toothpick should come out clean.

Dessert - Stuffed Dates

Ingredients:
Pitted dates
Natural peanut butter
Raisins
Chopped Nuts

What to do:
- Cute Fresh, pitted date in half.

- Stuff with natural peanut butter

- Top with raisins and nuts

- That's it. Simple, but delicious. I give these as gifts in a decorated metal tin.

Dessert - Sweet Potato Pie

Ingredients:
3/4 cup filtered water without fluoride
2 free-range chicken eggs (1 egg can be used.)
1/4 cup EVOO
3/4 cup raw honey
1/4 teaspoon ground cloves OR 2 or 3 whole cloves
1 teaspoon ground cinnamon
1/2 teaspoon ground ginger
1/2 teaspoon sea salt (See Index: Salt Example)
1-1/2 cups baked sweet potato (About 1 medium sweet potato –3/4 pound)

Topping: 1/2-to-3/4 cup Chopped or whole pecans

Pick a pie crust recipe from this book. Please see the Index at the back of the book:

What to do:
Preheat oven to 350 degrees:
In blender:
- Add water, eggs, EVOO, honey, cloves, cinnamon, ginger and salt.

- Add sweet potato half at a time and blend after each addition. (Mixture should be smooth.)

- Pour blender ingredients into finished pie crust.

- Sprinkle with 1/2 cup-to-3/4 cups of chopped or whole pecans on top. (make it look pretty)

- Bake at 350 degrees for 45 minutes.

NOTE:
Mixture should be about 4-1/2 cups in the blender when finished. If not, add more baked sweet potato.

Cook Ahead Mock Sausage Meat

Ingredients:
12 pounds non-hormone, free-range boneless, skinless chicken thigh meat or any non-hormone meat
3 cups filtered water without fluoride
3/4 cups of minced garlic
2 Tablespoons sea salt (See Index: Salt Example)
1 Tablespoon cayenne pepper
3 Tablespoons Italian Seasoning
1/4 cup EVOO

What to do:
- **Grind meat with meat grinder (I bought an electric meat grinder for about $100. Hand grinders cost less but require muscle power.)**

In Measuring Cup:
- **Blend with a spoon the water and minced garlic.**

In small bowl:
- **Blend with a spoon the salt, cayenne and Italian Seasoning.**

- **In 8 quart mixing bowl:**

- Add 12 pounds of ground meat.
- Add measuring cup and small bowl ingredients.
- Mix well with a rubber spatula.
- Cover with plastic wrap and let stand in the refrigerator overnight so spices can mingle together.
- After 8-to-10 hours; fry in iron skillet with 1/4 cup EVOO until cooked. Stir often and use your stainless steel utensil to cut meat. This will give a "crumbly" ground beef look. Let cool and divide into 12 freezer bags. Keeps for one-to-two months in the freezer.

Cook Ahead Meatloaf and 3 more meals

Ingredients:
Use 5 pounds total for five meals:
Mock Sausage (use 3 lbs meat of 5):
1 teaspoon sea salt (See Index: Salt Example)
1-1/2 Tablespoons Italian Seasoning
1 teaspoon cayenne pepper
3 pounds of non-hormone ground meat
6 Tablespoons minced garlic
1/2 cup filtered water without fluoride
Meatloaf Seasonings (use 2 lbs meat of 5 lbs.)
1 can beans, rinsed (Ingredients: beans, water, salt) OR Home-canned beans
1 medium onion (peeled and cut into quarters)
1 Tablespoon minced garlic
1/2 teaspoon cayenne pepper
1 cup old fashioned oatmeal (for the 2 lbs of meat for the meat loaf)

What to do:
Mock Sausage:
In small bowl:
- Add salt, Italian seasonings & cayenne pepper.

- Stir with spoon to blend.

In large bowl:
- Add three pounds from the five pounds of non-hormone meat.

- Add small bowl seasonings.

- Mix garlic and water together & add to meat.

- Let stand for at least two hours. If time is short, fry immediately until brown. (I let my meat mixture store in the refrigerator overnight so the spices can mingle.)

In an iron skillet:
- Brown and keep separate and crumbly, like cooked ground beef.

- Let cool and divide into three, one-quart freezer bags for freezing. This saves time during the week. One package accents the Spaghetti, Crock Chili or Red Beans and Rice.

- Meatloaf (the other two pounds)

In blender:
- Add rinsed beans, onion, minced garlic & cayenne.

- Blend well.

Mixing Bowl:
- Add two pounds of meat.

- Add oatmeal and blender ingredients.

- Mix with a rubber spatula until blended.

- Divide into two, one-pound baking loaves sprayed with EVOO.

- Bake at 350 degrees for one hour-to-one-hour and one half.

Cook Ahead Meatloaf II for Freezing

Ingredients:
1 cup filtered water without fluoride
1 quart cooked white beans
(four cups)—you must use fresh beans, not canned, for freezing—see bean recipe in this section
2 teaspoons sea salt (See Index: Salt Example)
1 teaspoon cayenne pepper
1 medium onion, peeled
1 Tablespoon of minced garlic
12 pounds non-hormone meat
(I grind my own chicken but turkey or beef works, too. Key words: "Free-range meat.")
4 cups old fashioned oatmeal

What to do:
In a blender:
- Blend water, beans, salt, pepper, onion and minced garlic until smooth.

In an 8 quart mixing bowl:
- Add meat, oatmeal and blender ingredients.

- Mix with rubber spatula or large spoon until blended.

- Spray EVOO into one-pound loaf pans. This should make about 12.

- Bake at 350 degrees for one hour-to one hour twenty minutes. I never have enough pans, so I must rotate the cooking, cooling and then reloading the pans to start the cycle over.

- Let cool. Take out of pans.

- Cut meatloaf into serving sizes so everyone gets a "Deck-of-cards" size piece.

- Put into freezer bags. Keeps for one-to-two months in the freezer.

Cook Ahead Shredded Chicken

Ingredients:
12 pounds of non-hormone OR sometimes called "Free-range" chicken breasts
2 Tablespoons homemade minced garlic

What to do:
In a large pot:
Boil chicken in enough filtered water without fluoride to cover.

Add two rounded Tablespoons of homemade minced garlic.

Boil until meat is white and flaky.

Shred two cups of the meat and wrap in wax paper. Then put into a quart freezer bag.

NOTE: I use this meat for the Chicken and Yellow Rice recipe, sandwiches in a Flatbread rolled up with vegetables. I home can or freeze the broth from boiling the chicken.

Dr. B's Recipe

This is my adapted Dr. B's Recipe (Batmanghelidj) for drinking every day.

- 1 quart glass jar (I use a Ball canning jar.)
- Fill the jar with filtered water without fluoride. Fluoride is a topical medicine for cavity prevention and should NOT be put inside your body. It would be like me drinking sun tan lotion to prevent my skin from burning at the beach.
- Add 1/4 teaspoon of coarse ground Celtic Sea Salt. (never table salt)
- Shake five or six times to add more oxygen and to help dissolve the salt.
- That's it. You're done.

We started our One Week Cleanse by drinking one quart of Dr. B's Recipe every day. For the second week, you may increase to two quarts of Dr. B's Recipe ONLY if you do NOT have any one of the following symptoms:

- The bags under your eyes have gotten larger or puffier.
- Your ankles and/or feet are swollen by day's end, but in the morning they are back to looking normal most of the time.
- Your stomach seems to be bloated much more than normal and it a little sensitive to the touch.
- You get sick to your stomach after drinking one quart of water and salt.
- Something in your inner self says, "No."

If you have only **one** symptoms mentioned above, then wait at **least** one more week before starting to drink the second quart of Dr. B's Recipe. Slow and steady wins the race.

Your end goal will be to drink 1/2 of your body weight each and every day. EXAMPLE: A 200 pound person will drink 100 ounces of filtered water without fluoride with approximately 1/4 teaspoon of Celtic sea salt per 32 ounces of water.

Home Canning Information

The "Ball" company offers a free cookbook for canning. It is by far the best bargain going. It is a full-color book. It is packed with information. The "Ball" company wants to encourage you to home can. Me, too.

Ball will give you their book and you pay for the shipping. It's where I go for all my canning information.

Here's how you can order your own copy: **1-800-240-3340**. They also sell "hard-to-find" supplies – like a stainless steel funnel made especially for canning.

My Frequent Canning Times:
Apple Butter:
Pints 10 minutes at 10 pounds of pressure

Beans:
Pints: 20 minutes at 10 pounds of pressure
Quarts: 25 minutes at 10 pounds of pressure

Chicken Stock
Pints: 20 minutes at 10 pounds of pressure
Quarts: 25 minutes at 10 pounds of pressure

Spaghetti Sauce
Pints: 35 minutes at 10 pounds of pressure
Quarts 40 minutes at 10 pounds of pressure

Cook Ahead Beans

Cook Ahead White Beans/Pinto Beans or "Whatever" Beans for Canning or Freezing

What to do:
All beans (red, white, pinto, black etc.) basically cook the same:
In a 5-1/2 quart Crock Pot:

- 4-1/2 cups dry beans

- Wash and pick bad ones out

- Add 6 cups of filtered water without fluoride.

- Add 8 cups of boiling hot water. If the water isn't boiling, this may not work!

- 1 Tablespoon minced garlic

- 1 teaspoon sea salt

- You will want to add more water so there is a ½ inch of empty space at the top of the crock pot before the lid. This makes the beans have some sauce. You'll put some of the sauce over the beans into each jar. Use a wooden spoon to stir the beans in the jar to remove any air pockets. The canning book will give you exact instructions.

- **Put on the lid and set the crock pot to low heat over night (Eight-to-ten hours)**

Freezing Note:
 If you don't have the equipment to home can, you can freeze this recipe in a glass jar with a tight-fitting lid. WARNING: Leave one inch of head room (air space at the top of the jar) to give your ingredients room to expand without breaking the glass jar.

 Makes 8 pints. Each pint is equal to a can of store-bought beans.

Snack - Bean Sprouts

Ingredients:
* Glass Jar
* Mesh bag approximately 3 inches wide by 8 inches high. I made a bag from a woven laundry bag with holes. The holes are like a large cloth weave. I bought it at the Dollar Store. You can buy a sprouting bag, but I didn't want to wait for it to be delivered—and they are rather pricey.
* Dry lentil beans

What to do:
In a glass jar (I use a Quart Canning Jar.)
- **Add 3/4 cup of dry lentil beans**

- **Cover with filtered water without fluoride.**

- **Let sit on the kitchen counter over night to soak (No need to cover jar.)**

<u>**Here's the Process:**</u>

- I divided the laundry bag into four smaller bags and then sewed the bags on my sewing machine. Each bag is approximately 9" by 12".

- Pour the lentils into one of these bags after soaking overnight or buy a "spouting bag."

- I rinse the beans for ten-to-fifteen seconds under my filtered water without fluoride spout.

- I hung the bag from a kitchen cabinet door to start.

- Later I bought a banana tree—to hang bananas from. Put a dish underneath to catch any dripping water. Nice. It has a permanent home on my counter.

- Put a dish under the bag to catch the excess water.

- At bedtime, I give the beans their shower. (Rinse with filtered water without fluoride.)

Next morning, I give them another shower.
- At night I repeat and give them another shower.

- Not a lot of time for the cook, but since the bag is on my counter, I do see it all the time so I can remember to give them their quickie shower.

- Finally, on the third day—you have sprouts.

- If the beans miss one shower, not a bigee. These are yummy and addictive.

- I remove the sprouts from the bag.

- Store in a glass quart jar in the refrigerator.

- **Put the lid on, and the sprouts stay for four or five days in the refrigerator.**

- **Sometimes I put them in a plastic bag for an on-the go snack. Tasty on salads and sandwiches, too.**

Replenish Friendly Germs in your Gut. Beans are the perfect food to add to your diet. A good source of protein and a wonderful source of fiber. There's lots of healthy flora on this food because you grow it right in your own kitchen on top of your counter-top farm. Fiber, according to David Reuben, M.D. is a key factor in preventing colon cancer! I use lentil beans. They are tiny and make wonderful sprouts.

Snack - Popcorn

Air-popped popcorn WAS a great snack. Why "was?" In 2014, I bought a Presto air popper and after three consecutive days of using it, I had a headache. I was shocked. Did I examine the popper machine before the headache? I am ashamed to say, "No."

When the popper came out of the box, it smelled like plastic, horrible plastic! The chute where the un-popped kernels go looked like four inches of aluminum. I are dumb. No wonder I got a headache with all that plastic! A BPA free popper may be better, but I cannot find any that don't use aluminum for the popcorn chute.

Ingredients for two servings:
1 cup popping corn, I use "Jollytime."
Sea salt (See Index: Salt Example)

1/2 cup EVOO (extra virgin olive oil)

What to do:
For two servings:
- **Make sure the skillet is NOT larger than the burner.**

- **On medium heat let the skillet heat up for five minutes. I use a timer or I have tried to burn the house down.**

- **Add the EVOO and popcorn in the center of the skillet. Give it a stir so all of the popcorn kernels are covered in the EVOO.**

- **Put on the lid. (a glass lid works nice so I can see the cooking progression of the popcorn.**

- **When you hear the first POP POP, start to push the skillet up and back on the burner. Hold down the lid with one hand, as you gently move the pan up and back. This takes about three minutes of babysitting.**

- **When the popping is only one every five seconds, your popcorn is done otherwise you start to burn the popcorn. Remove from the heat and serve.**

- **Sprinkle sea salt and stir using a spoon. This is HOT! Please use a spoon.**

Popcorn Popper Review: I tried the stainless steel popcorn maker with the handle that turns the popcorn in the oil at the bottom, and it worked okay. I do NOT recommend this because the clean up time is HORRIBLE! I like the iron skillet method best.

Easy clean up and I already own the skillet. The skillet should be the size of your burner for even heat.

I have also tried this with a glass pot that has a lid, and it works good. I like it slightly better than the iron skillet because I can see the popcorn popping. The bad side is that the clean up time can be longer when you burn the popcorn. I still miss my air popper, but I do NOT miss the headache I received from it.

Final winning score: Iron skillet. I use the glass lid with the iron skillet, and it is easy to use and fun to watch.

Snack - Popcorn Treat

Ingredients:
1/2 cup raw honey
1/4 cup EVOO (extra virgin olive oil)
2 cups dry roasted peanuts (no salt)
8 cups of popped popcorn from the above recipe, but do NOT add salt.

What to do:
In a fry pan.
- **Heat honey and EVOO until warm.**
- **Add nuts and stir to coat nuts.**
- **Add four cups of popcorn .**
- **Stir until popcorn is coated.**

In a 12 X 9 glass baking dish:

- Add the other four cups of popcorn on the bottom of dish.
- Use a rubber spatula to remove mixture from fry pan.
- Pour fry pan mixture on top of popcorn in baking dish.
- Bake at 300 degrees for 5 minutes.
- Stir. Bake 5 more minutes.
- Stir and bake 5 more minutes. (15 minutes total)
- Let cool on wax paper on a cookie rack. Then peel off wax paper to store in baggies for individual servings or in a glass bowl with a lid. Will stay fresh in the refrigerator for about a week.

Nut Yogurt (Yoghurt)

You may think I have paranoia, because I prefer NOT to purchase organic yogurt or sour cream. Why? I simply try to avoid trusting Food Manufacturers as much as I possibly can. This is an excellent way to eat your probiotics or friendly germs without a pill. See the index to find out why you want to eat your germs every day. Find: "friendly germs are responsible for."

Ingredients:
Filtered water without fluoride
1 cup of RAW cashews
1 Tablespoon Grade A Maple Syrup

What to do:
In a glass quart canning jar:
- **Place nuts in jar.**

- Add about two cups of filtered water without fluoride. Nuts must be covered by the water.

- Cover jar with a paper towel and rubber band the paper towel to the jar or use the glass ring of a canning jar.

- Let soak overnight (8-to-12 hours)

In a blender in the morning:
- Drain water.

- Add half cup of water, cashews and maple syrup.

- Blend until creamy. The consistency looks like yogurt. Add a little more water if too difficult to blend or too thick.

- Put on the lid and store in the refrigerator.

- Stays fresh for at least a week. You'll know it is bad because it doesn't smell pleasant.

Serving Suggestion: Use as you would yogurt or sour cream. I love this on the burrito, a wrap, a bread dip, baked potato, fruit smoothie or on top of my Lazy Bread.

Snack Choices

Important Goal!! Eat Five Small Meals a Day

Pick Two Snacks Every day (NOT an option) This will increase liver function. 10:00 a.m. Snack and 3:00 p.m. Snack

- Apples (An Apple a Day Does Keep the Doctor Away)
- Celery or Carrots (with peanut butter?)
- Homemade Cucumbers (cut into spears. Optional: peeled)
- Pickles (without alum, colorings or sodium benzoate.)
- All the fresh fruit you can eat!
- Frozen or fresh Grapes
- Melons
- Figs (not in a package)
- Nuts (salt is okay, roasted without oil)
- Seeds (sunflower and other varieties)
- Raisins (box for easy carrying. Ingredients: California seedless raisins)
- Peanut butter (ingredients: peanuts)
- Whole wheat bread (no crackers with enriched flour or hydrogenated oil)
- Apple butter (from this cookbook) on roll or bread)
- Popcorn (from the recipe in this book)

- Cherry tomatoes

- Anything leftover from this cookbook

- Mock Cracker Jacks

- Salad & EVOO Salad Dressing

- Cinnamon Buns from this cookbook

- Organic dairy maximum is 3 - Half cup servings a week.

- Lazy Bread, toasted.

- Lazy Bread with peanut butter and apple butter recipe from this book.

Drink Choices

Number One Choice: Water and Salt or Dr. B's Recipe. (See Index) We started our One Week Cleanse by drinking one quart of Dr. B's Recipe every day. For the second week, you may increase to two quarts of Dr. B's Recipe ONLY if you do NOT have any one of the following symptoms:

- The bags under your eyes have gotten larger or puffier.
- Your ankles and/or feet are swollen by day's end, but in the morning they are back to looking normal most of the time.
- Your stomach seems to be bloated much more than normal and it slightly hurts to the touch.
- You get sick to your stomach after drinking one quart of water and salt.
- Something in your inner self says, "No."

If you have only **one** symptoms mentioned above, then wait at least one more week before starting to drink the second quart of Dr. B's Recipe. Slow and steady wins the race.

Your goal in two or three months will be to drink 1/2 of your body weight each and every day. EXAMPLE: A 200 pound person will drink 100 ounces of filtered water without fluoride with approximately 1/4 teaspoon of Celtic sea salt per 32 ounces of water.

You can drink coffee or other caffeine drink, but for every cup you drink you must drink THREE additional cups of water to replace the water that was removed from your body.

Promoting Digestion:

Herbal Peppermint tea –hot or cold is a great drink to help your stomach produce the right ratio of digestive juices to promote digestion. (there isn't any caffeine in peppermint tea.) Better digestion helps weight loss. Drink as often as you like because it doesn't have caffeine. Make sure you check the ingredient's label before you buy any tea. The label should say: peppermint leaves. That's it! Please, no black tea or flavorings.

Apple cider vinegar promotes digestion. 1 teaspoon in eight ounces of water. Take 20 minutes before you eat. Easier/faster digestion will promote gentle weight loss because you are detoxifying your body.

Kidney stones or bladder problems: Corn silk tea will dissolve your kidney stones and promote detoxification. Yes, you read that correctly! You can drink corn silk tea hot or cold. Sweeten with raw honey.

Drink - Corn silk tea recipe

Buy some raw corn with the husks still on them. I use two ears. Use the corn's tender leaves nearest the ear and the silk for the tea.

- Boil 8 cups of filtered water without fluoride. Then place the silk into water. Continue to cook on low-to-medium heat for about 15 minutes.
- Take off the heat and cover with a tight-fitting lid. Let stand at least 20 minutes. Strain and your tea is ready. Stays in the fridge for about a week.

My son-in-law was diagnosed as a "chronic stone former." He drank two cups of this tea and his water requirement nonstop for six months and reported that he easily passed over 10 stones. As a way to keep himself clear of future problems, he drinks two cups of tea once a month for three or four days. He said, "I would hear a "plop" in the toilet bowl and knew I had painlessly passed another stone!"

The tea "alone" will NOT produce these results. Dane also stopped eating the "Liver enemies" found in most food. The combination of no "Liver enemies," drinking his water requirement of half his body weight, and this tea, produced these results.

Depression & other emotional symptoms:

Because Food Manufacturers remove B vitamins in order to increase their food's shelf life, you may have a shortage that could contribute to depression & other emotional symptoms. To replenish your body's B Vitamins, drink unsulphured blackstrap molasses.

Why Blackstrap Molasses is good:

Blackstrap molasses is the third boiling of the sugar cane plant or sugar beet plant produces a thick dark syrup. Blackstrap molasses contains all the minerals, B vitamins and iron that was removed from making white refined sugar.

This is the main reason for sugar being so deadly to the human body. It is NOT that sugar is empty calories – NO! It is that sugar is an unbalanced food that produces a human that has unbalanced health. When sugar is eaten, the body is sent into a panic trying to balance white refined sugar. No nutrients. No vitamins. No iron and no way to digest the sugar. Your body sends sugar to the liver because it thinks it is a poison. Is it a poison? Yes, your body is correct. Sugar feeds cancer.

Unsulphered blackstrap molasses is sold in natural food stores for its nutritional benefits. It contains B vitamins, minerals and has iron. I put one tablespoon of unsulphered blackstrap molasses in a cup of hot water as a coffee substitute. It has a slightly bitter taste that takes a little getting used to, but it supplies that energy I want first thing in the morning.

I are dumb:

"Grandma's Molasses" is NOT blackstrap molasses. Yes, it is dark. Yes, they have an "unsulphered" variety, BUT it ain't the same. I was fooled by this product. When I emailed the company to ask if it was "blackstrap molasses," I never received a reply. I did some added research on the types of molasses – yes, there are three types: Who could have guessed?

1) Lite molasses. I am very suspicious when I see on the front of any label "lite." When Food Manufacturers make up food names with different spelling, I make a mad dash for an exit.

2) Dark molasses

3) Blackstrap molasses

Sheesh! I are dumb. I are trusting. Being an informed consumer takes a lot of work! BUT, in work's defense, it is worth it because I won't eat poison for my liver. The blackstrap has two different categories, too:

1) sulphered

2) unsulphered.

Whew! I could call this "trickery," but I know that it has NOTHING to do with trickery. This is just plain good marketing and business techniques. Bottom line for any business is to increase PROFITS – it just makes sense. What makes sense for us is to become educated.

I suggest, Unsulphered, Blackstrap Molasses and nothing else.

Drink Dandelion Tea

I grow my dandelions in a pot on my patio. The leaves and flowers from the dandelion plant are excellent for detoxifying! Did you think those weeds were worthless? God put a lot of dandelions on earth because He knew we would need a lot of cleaning up from our toxic world.

The leaves can be dried or just follow the same recipe as the corn silk tea recipe and substitute the corn leaves with dandelion leaves. Mix half tea, half 100% juice.

Water:

The disadvantages of using tap water for a drinking are environmental pollutants. According to 1990 Consumer Reports there are three drinking water pollutants of most concern. They are lead, radon and nitrates. Also, tap water has some minerals and chemicals added for "purification" purposes, including chlorine, alum or sodium aluminum salts, soda, ash, phosphates, calcium hydroxide and activated carbon. Not healthy!

Filtered water without fluoride:

Use the filtered water without fluoride for cooking and drinking. A reverse osmosis filter is the best water filter money can buy in my opinion and is the only filter that I know will removed fluoride. If this filter is not properly maintained, then it won't work. I prefer the filtered water without fluoride for more control over what goes in my body.

Wine or Grape Juice Basics

Paul wrote in the Bible that a little wine is good for the stomach. Finding wine the way Paul drank it in the 21st century is difficult—might be impossible. Why? Because Food

Manufacturers need their product wine to be cheap and fast. How do they accomplish this task? By using chemicals to "force" the natural fermenting process of the grapes to hurry up.

Chemicals are our health's enemy. If I drink processed wine, I get a dull headache the next day. I always thought the headache was caused by something blooming. I live in Florida, and plants blooming is "normal" here.

I did a little experimenting, and low and behold my dull headache was the wine. To me a dull, sinus-type headache the next day it is not worth a glass of wine the night before.

My remedy? I drink a glass of this fermented wine that I process on my kitchen counter. No dull headache. I drink a glass at night before bed. It is so tasty that it is difficult to believe that it is good for my health.

Grape Soda or Grape Wine

Ferment the grapes for 12 to 36 hours. (Depending on the temperature in your kitchen will determine how long the fermentation process takes. The way you tell when the grapes are great for a grape soda is by tasting.

When the taste is the way you like it, then strain all the grapes and put the drink into the refrigerator to stop the fermentation process. If you want wine, the same steps are taken to make grape soda, but the time on the kitchen counter is longer. Again, tasting is the only way to know when the wine is done. If you wait too long, you will have vinegar. Wine vinegar can be used for the salad dressing by removing the apple cider vinegar and replacing with your homemade vinegar.

Ingredients:
4 pounds ORGANIC grapes = see warning below (weight on the vine) almost eight quarts of filtered water without fluoride
- Eight, Quart Mason Jars: Less than $1 each when you buy twelve in a box

- <u>The formula:</u> Half pound of grapes per quart jar. Do not fill each jar to the top with water. Give about one inch to an inch and a half of head room for each jar.

What to do:
- **Evenly divide washed grapes taken off the bunch of grapes into eight Mason jars. Process each jar separately in the blender. You WON'T puree the water and grapes. You will pulse the blender to make a chunky mixture of grapes and water. This mixture would look like what you would imagine would happen if you took off your shoes and stomped the grapes with your feet – your clean feet.**

- **Return the chunky grape mixture to the quart jar.**

- **Add more filtered water without fluoride and give 1-1/2 inches of head room. This mixture expands when it ferments.**

- **On each jar put a paper towel on top. You can use the canning ring to hold the paper towel in place. (one or two twists of the ring should do it. Do not insert the canning insert for now.)**

- **Label the jars. with a date 48 hours in the future.**

- **Check taste in 48 hours. This makes a great sweet soda for children. If you want wine, let it ferment 72 hours longer and taste again.**

- **Taste test after another 12 hours. Sometimes you need another 24 hours for a better-tasting wine. When it tastes the way you like: 1) sweet 2) smells like wine, then strain the grapes and keep the liquid.**

- **Store in a pantry or on the kitchen counter top. When the cooler weather happens, these times may change. The grapes can be tossed in the garbage.**

- **Store your wine in the refrigerator – this will stop the fermenting process. If you let the grapes ferment longer, eventually you will get wine vinegar. This vinegar can be substituted for the Apple Cider Vinegar in the EVOO Salad Dressing. Yummy for adults.**

Grapes Warning:

Most grapes are prepackaged in a bag – keep your eyes wide open to read the small print on these bags. The print is miniscule and says something like: "Treated with sulphur dioxide for fungicide use. "

Wikipedia says, "a colorless pungent toxic gas formed by burning sulfur in the air." Yes, this is a preservative, disinfectant and BLEACH that is used to make sulfuric acid. That's the long form – the short form? Liver enemy. This preservative is responsible for people with asthma to have an attack or for others – like me – to have a headache.

If you cannot find grapes that have not been sprayed, skip this recipe. Also, take caution not to serve grape soda that has been fermenting over 48 hours to a child. You can smell the difference between grape soda and grape wine. If the drink smells like wine, it is wine. The alcohol content is very, very low, (less than one percent) but should always be a consideration when making this fermented drink.

Substitutes for Recipes

Cocoa (Hot)

1 Tablespoon Baker's Cocoa
1-to-2 Tablespoons Raw Honey
Pinch of cinnamon
2 or 3 shakes of Black Pepper (optional)
1 cup hot filtered water without fluoride
Mix and enjoy.

Chinese Mustard

In very small bowl, put a small amount of dry mustard. (two teaspoons) Add 5-or-6 drops of filtered water without fluoride to the dry mustard. Make a light paste of dry mustard powder with the filtered water without fluoride. This is very spicy – - even a little hot to some. Good for dipping.

Garlic Oil or Garlic EVOO

When you don't have three days to wait.

- 1/4 cup EVOO plus one level teaspoon of minced garlic.
- Hot Spiced Apple Tea:
- Heat one cup 100% apple juice. Add a pinch of ground cinnamon and a drop of lemon juice or apple cider vinegar.

Which is better for your health? Lard or Margarine?

Never use any other cooking oil than Extra Virgin Olive Oil. Never, ever use margarine. Why? It is not food. Lard is a better choice for your health than margarine! And everyone knows how bad lard is for your health. But Lard is a natural product that is made from food, while Margarine is NOT natural but man-made and that is the real sign of a way to poison your health. Put another way? Margarine is man-made food and therefore—POISON!

Lemon Peel Tea:

Please use a lemon that hasn't had pesticides put on it.

- Don't discard lemon skins after using the juice. Lemon skin should be washed well.
- Put 1/4 lemon peel in cup of hot water.
- Let steep for 5 minutes.
- Remove lemon peel.
- Sweeten to taste with raw honey.

Lemonade Mix

Into a two-quart jug:

- Squeeze two medium to large fresh lemons.
- Add 2-to-3 Tablespoons of Grade A maple syrup, or raw honey
- Add filtered water without fluoride to fill container.

- Shake, chill and serve.

Mock Baking Powder

BEWARE! Baking Powder has aluminum! A bad choice. Researchers say that aluminum contributes to Alzheimer's Disease.

- **For recipes that call for one teaspoon of Baking Powder use 1 ½ teaspoons of Apple Cider vinegar plus 1 teaspoon baking soda.**

NOTE:

All purpose flour has NO PURPOSE! Don't eat it. It depletes from your family's health and contributes to tooth decay.

Mock Cream (for cooking

In a Blender:

- **1/2 cup filtered water without fluoride**
- **2 Tablespoons whole-wheat flour**
- **2 Tablespoons EVOO**
- **1 teaspoon raw honey**
- **Blend until smooth. Can be used for mashed potatoes. If you want garlic mashed potatoes, replace the 2 Tablespoons of EVOO with garlic EVOO.**

Mock Milk (for cooking

or use the Almond Milk recipe in this book.

Ingredients:
1 Tablespoon EVOO (extra virgin olive oil)
1 cup filtered water without fluoride
1 Tablespoon raw honey or Grade A Maple Syrup

What to do:
- **Stir and use.**

Mock Lemon Juice

Apple Cider Vinegar substitutes very nicely instead of lemon juice in most recipes.

Mock White Sugar (in recipes

Replace one cup of white sugar with 3/4 cup of honey and eliminate 1/4 cup liquid from the recipe. If there isn't a place to reduce the liquid, add 3 Tablespoons of whole wheat flour.

- **Use grade A maple syrup. Use 1-1/3 cup of maple syrup and eliminate 1/4 cup liquid from the recipe.**

- **Use 1-1/4 cup unsulphered black strap molasses. Also, add 1/4 cup of whole wheat flour to the recipe. (Be careful: Black strap molasses has its own "distinctive" taste.)**

Meat Recommendations

Keep your portion of meat to about 15-to-20 percent of your entire meal. Eat meat two times a day MAXIMUM. The older I become, the less meat I eat because I trust Food Manufacturers less and less each year as I see them manipulate food ingredient labels MORE AND MORE.

Eating meat about the size of a deck of cards is recommended. Eat meat as an accent and NOT the entire meal. Eating less meat is easier for your digestion. Easier digestion means easier weight management and quicker healing.

Hormones in your food has been linked to heart disease and stroke along with other illnesses. Please know that many of the foods in this book have protein in them and NO meat.

The Protein Myth:

A baked potato is equal in protein as mother's milk. Mother's milk can take a limp new born that cannot turn over in bed, into a one year old little wild Indian climbing onto any and all furniture.

People in Bible days strictly ate meat for religious holidays and special occasions. That equates to eating meat about a half dozen times a YEAR! B12 – that is found in meat can be re-circulated in the human body for three or four months.

Please don't buy into the protein myth that you must eat protein in order to make muscle. It is a myth – just ask a gorilla that doesn't eat meat.

The protein myth is fueled by Food Manufacturers that sell protein powders. Protein powders are NOT healthy. One of my students ate a protein shake every day for body building, and suffered with horrible neck and joint pain. He stopped the protein powder and his joint pain decreased.

Substitutes More

Ants: Cream of Tartar repels ants. This is a chemical, and should NOT be used in your food.

Bug Bites

Apple Cider Vinegar helps relieve itching of a bug bite.

- Inflammation or redness can be help with Garlic Oil:

Baby Powder or Foot Powder:

Cornstarch

- Use cornstarch instead of baby or foot powder. This is a fragrance and chemical free alternative.
- Cornstarch repels roaches. (don't eat cornstarch)
- Cornstarch freshens carpets. 1) Sprinkle on carpet. 2) Brush in (optional) 3) Wait 30 minutes. 4) Vacuum.
- Cornstarch is NOT to thicken soups. Because it is processed food. Use whole wheat flour instead: 1) Dissolve whole wheat flour in a little water or cooled broth before adding to gravies or soups. 2) Stir in with spoon. This method avoids lumps.

Deodorant

I use a deodorant stone. Yes, it works. Make sure your deodorant doesn't have aluminum in it. Aluminum can be absorbed through the skin, and is linked with Alzheimer's Disease. I've read that baking soda is another alternative that can be used by applying a little under the arms.

Drain Cleaner

Put baking soda down the drain (1 or 2 Tablespoons.) Then pour a few cups of white vinegar into the drain until it starts to bubble. This may take two or three applications to completely unclog a bad clog, but will improve with each application.

Drain Freshener

Combine one cup of white vinegar with two quarts of boiling water. Pour down drain.

Gargle

Mix 1/2 cup filtered water without fluoride with 1/2 cup Apple Cider Vinegar. For laryngitis or sore throat, gargle every two hours.

Hair Dye Warning

According to "Living Healthy in a Toxic World" by David Steinman, lead acetate in men's hair dye is absorbed through the skin and is dangerous.

Also, avoid using any product with the word "P-phenylenediamine" on the ingredients label. This chemical is dangerous. Never dye your hair when pregnant, to protect the unborn baby.

Yes, I dye my hair. I use Pure Indigo Leaf Powder (no PPD) and Henna. 2 Tablespoons of Indigo to 2 Tablespoon of Henna for dark brown hair color. I do not have a suggestion for other colors. See my website for more information.

Hair Frizzes

- 1 Tablespoon honey
- 2 teaspoons EVOO
- Mix and apply to hair.
- Wrap head in warm towel for 20 minutes.
- Shampoo.

Mock Play Dough

- 2 cups all-purpose flour
- 1 cup iodized salt or regular salt
- 1 teaspoon cream of tartar (never eat this)
- 2 Tablespoon oil
- Stir over medium heat for three minutes.
- Knead to right consistency.

Paper Mache

- 1 cup flour
- 2/3 cup water
- Combine.
- Dip strips of newspaper and use.

Stainless Steel Cleaner:

Cloth dampened with white vinegar. Or spray directly on stainless steel and wipe off with a dry rag.

Tile Cleaner:

I use white vinegar at full strength. It cleans grout that looks black! Use a brush to scrub the black away. The black is sometimes mold, and vinegar kills mold.

Window & Counter Top Cleaner:

50/50 mix: Half white vinegar to half water. This window cleaner kills germs and doesn't streak.

Herbal Liver Medicine – Milk Thistle

I suggest that you try this herbal remedy ONLY after you have been drinking filtered water without fluoride for at least a month AND you have been successful eating this diet for at least a month, too.

Just doing the herbal remedy and forgetting the other suggestions in this book is NOT recommended.

Ingredient of what you need:

- *"Organic Milk Thistle" in their whole form.* <u>http://www.migrainephd.com/love-your-liver/</u>
- *One bottle of 100 proof Vodka - 700 ml in a <u>glass</u> bottle. I bought this at a local liquor store.*
- *One glass jar and lid (64 ounces) I used an empty raw honey jar.)*
- *One empty glass bottle that has a glass dropper. I used an old tincture bottle that was washed and relabeled.*

What to do:
In the quart jar:
- **Add one cup of Milk Thistle herb into the 64 ounce glass jar.**
- **Add the entire Vodka bottle contents.**
- **Cover with a tight-fitting lid.**
- **Let it sit out on the kitchen counter for six weeks.**

- **I gave it a gentle shake every morning.**

- **At the end of the six weeks, I use a large strainer to remove the Milk Thistle herb and what is left is a dark herbal liquid remedy that is called, "milk thistle tincture."**

- **Transfer some of the tincture into a small, glass bottle that has a glass dropper. Store the leftovers in a glass jar, and store it in a dark cabinet.**

- **I suggest starting with one drop of the tincture into a glass of filtered water without fluoride every morning. This is an herbal remedy and will not send you to the hospital for a little more or a little less. If I use too much, I will get a dull headache as a warning sign from my body. Why the headache? Because I am pushing my body to detoxify too quickly. NOT a good choice. If you get a head ache, stop use for one week. Continue ONLY eating from this book, and revisit taking the herb.**

- **After a week, you may want to increase your dosage to 7 drops – up to one dropper full. (You be the judge.)**

This remedy will not grow stale or become unusable to my knowledge. Milk thistle is one of the most-researched herbs for its liver rejuvenating properties.

Planning a Simple Party

An easy party favorite would be pizza or the chili Most people I know love pizza. Make the spaghetti sauce early in the week. The day of the party prepare the salsa for chips (chip ingredients say: corn & salt) or celery and carrot sticks to dip. This dip is used for Mexican eggs, too.

The pizza dough can be made on the morning of the party and rolled out when you are ready to assemble the pizza. The party menu might look like this:

1) Chips (Ingredients say: corn & salt) with Salsa or veggies on the side.

2) Mexican Eggs

3) Pizza

4) Hot Popcorn (The smell also adds to a "fun" atmosphere.)

5) How about a walk around the neighborhood? badminton in the yard?? If the weather doesn't allow, how about a game of war with a deck of cards? Don't under estimate the goodness of simple pleasures.

Addendum: 21 Ways to Love Your Liver for a Healthier you!

There must be 50 ways to love your liver – or is that leave your lover? Hmmm. Well, here are 21 ways to get you on your way to feeling better with a healthier liver. First and foremost,

PLEASE do not rush through these steps because I designed them to be baby steps. That means take it slow. My suggestion is to do one liver treatment per week. If you are really sick, take one liver treatment per month. It is important to do the steps.

Please remember:

Slow and steady wins the race!

Liver Treatment One

Remove all fake sweeteners and related products that contain man-made sweeteners from your house!

Replace all the sweet in your house to be raw honey or grade A Maple syrup. Pile it on. Honey helps your immune system and will satisfy your sweet tooth.

100 percent of my students who ate fake sugar never gained one pound when they stopped eating it. Not one. Why? Because it

is all a LIE promoted by profits! Food Manufacturers want to sell their food to another market – the people who want to lose weight – would that be you? Stop it. Stop it NOW.

Liver Treatment Two

Eat one serving of fresh, raw fruit each day.

Eat a serving is equal to about one cup.

Eating one serving of your favorite RAW fruit each day will have many health benefits for a happier liver:

- Adds fiber for constipation relief. If have diarrhea, you still need to eat RAW fruit to fix your bowel health problem. Try to eat one or two RAW bananas. (Until the diarrhea stops completely.)

- Friendly bacteria is a part of all raw fruits and will help repopulate your gut with good bacteria and helps with constipation and diarrhea, too.

- Satisfies any cravings for sweet in a healthy method.

- Helps normalize blood sugar levels.

- Fruit will increase your energy so you can do some of the things you love to do.

Liver Treatment Three

Eat your second serving of fresh, raw fruit every day.

A serving is equal to about one cup.

Eating two servings of fruit each day will have many health benefits for a happier liver:

- Helps to repopulate friendly bacteria in the gut. The friendly bacteria will help with constipation and/or diarrhea.

- Fruit is a fast breakfast.

- Fruit is great to eat anytime. Eat your fruit for a 10:00 a.m. snack and then a 3:00 p.m. snack.

- If you have diarrhea, please focus eating your raw fruit as a banana or two bananas TWICE a day.

- If you are hungry right before bed, eat a serving of fruit.

- No, it won't cause you to have nightmares or keep you up because fruit is easy to digest.

- No, it won't put on extra weight on your body because eating a raw sweet right before bed is easy to digest. Fruit has all of the enzymes to digest itself – unlike processed, white sugar.

- So, what is the bottom line for the best time of day to eat your two servings of fruit? Are you guessing? If you said, "Anytime is the best time." You were correct. Your goal? **EAT THE FRUIT!**

Liver Treatment Four

Eat a raw salad every day for one complete meal.

This is really a HUGE step because changing one meal every day will result in big statistics towards a happy liver. What do I mean? Think of it this way, you will change 1/3 of your eating habits by just changing one meal each day. That is pretty impressive for just beginning to read this book.

What should you eat in your salad? Only fresh, raw veggies. This is the best way to add more friendly bacteria to your body that will balance your gut very quickly.

Friendly bacteria live on and in all fresh fruits and vegetables and is beneficial to your liver. After a week of just doing this little, tiny step you should begin to feel better. Your first SIMPLE recipe.

Don't panic. Take a deep breath and read it before your throw your hands up in defeat:

<u>Simple Salad Dressing:</u>

- ½ cup Apple Cider Vinegar
- ¾ cup EVOO (extra virgin olive oil)

You may add Celtic sea salt at the table. This recipe may seem a little plain but simple is the best way to start your new path to happiness. The apple cider vinegar will begin to detoxify you, and the EVOO is helping your liver to get the healthy fat that it so desperately needs to encourage you to improved liver function.

What is an unhealthy fat? Margarine and vegetable oil are two of the most popular bad fats. STOP it! EVOO is the only fat you may eat until you start to feel better.

When you eat this salad, please fill up. Don't worry about gaining weight because it never, ever happens to any of my students.

How much dressing should you use?

Backstroke!

Eat as much as you like! This is food as medicine. Enjoy it! NO! You won't gain weight. Trust me! You will feel better – don't argue.

The most difficult part will be the shopping, but the next hardest part will be allotting enough time for you to chew all of the raw veggies. (Get your helper to chop the veggies.)

A Note about eating at a salad bar:

Two main rules:

1) Just eat RAW
2) bring your own homemade salad dressing from home. (the simple recipe above is all you should eat until you start to feel better.)

Salad bar no – no's:

- DON'T eat mushrooms swimming in an unknown sauce.
- DON'T add pickles that have been swimming in a juice.

- DON'T eat crunchy bacon bits that are usually man-made something.

- DON'T eat croutons. They have not been fried in a healthy oil.

- DON'T eat meat, cheese, yogurt, cottage cheese or other foods made from animal products because these foods are usually filled with hormones and contribute to liver disease.

- What is the keyword here? R-A-W, raw and whole foods.

Will you be hungry a few hours after eating the salad because you body is so happy and digesting your food quickly? You bet! You will be **STARVING**! Yes, out of your mind hungry – crazy – give me FOOD! Give me Food **NOW**! Yay! What's the answer?

I use a baby bottle to carry my salad dressing into the restaurant with me. I put the baby bottle into a plastic baggie so it will catch any drips that might ruin my purse.

Liver Treatment Five

Eat a cracker and peanut butter for breakfast

What kind of peanut butter? Ingredients: peanuts – that's it. What kind of cracker? If you cannot find this name brand cracker or one with similar ingredients, then skip this Liver Treatment. Yes, it is very important that you eat a simple cracker with the exact ingredients.

WASA Ingredients:

Front of the label it says:

Wasa, baked since 1919

Light rye crisp bread

Bloating warning:

Only eat one cracker because they are extremely high in fiber. Too much fiber too fast may cause bloating or gas. Remember, the goal in this book is to start slow and move slow. Success will be yours when you keep marching forward with the Liver Treatments in this book. If you hate this cracker, skip this treatment.

Liver Treatment Six

Replace all the fats in your house to EVOO.

What does the word "fats" mean?

If you use vegetable oil for cooking, stop. If you use soybean oil, stop. You may not eat margarine anymore. You may not eat any other fat but EVOO. EVOO is short for "extra virgin olive oil."

- No butter
- no mayonnaise
- no mustard.

- no yogurt
- no cream

Fat you must use:

1. Mock mayo.
2. Mock EVOO mustard.
3. Peanut butter only ingredient: roasted peanuts or use the recipe in this book.

If you cannot make the three fats suggested above, then go cold turkey until you start to feel better and can devote some time to cooking in your own kitchen. My main advice I want you to hear is:

Move Slow!

YOU MUST EAT GOOD FAT!

Remove the bad fats from your kitchen and put them in another part of the house where you won't accidentally cook with them.

Liver Treatment Seven

Eat an avocado for breakfast

The high good fat content of the avocado and the high vitamin A content both contribute to it being a liver's super food. If you can, eat at least two or three avocados a week. I prefer the variety of avocado called, "Haas." It has a little more flavorful taste than the avocado locally grown here in Florida. Any variety of avocado you can find will do just fine.

How to pick an avocado:

The avocado must be somewhat hard to the squeeze. The more it gives, the riper it is. I do NOT like an extremely soft or an extremely hard avocado. A subtle giving of the fruit says, "I'm ready to eat."

I usually buy a few avocados at a time that are rock hard. These avocados will ripen on my kitchen counter. Every morning they receive a squeeze from me to check out if today is the day I get to eat one of them.

If it ripens faster than I thought, I put it into the refrigerator to buy some time before I am ready to eat it. A ripe avocado will usually last two or three days in the refrigerator after it has ripened and won't become rotten.

What to do:
- Cut the avocado length wise from where the stem was and all around to where you started. You won't be able to cut the avocado in half because there is a very large pit in the center.

- Pull the two halves apart with your fingers.

- Sprinkle a little Celtic sea salt on it.

- Get your spoon and eat it like the skin was your bowl.

- Remove the pit and eat the second half with your spoon, too.

An avocado is a very simple and delicious breakfast. High in vitamin A and it will help populate your friendly bacteria as well as boost your energy because your liver will say, "thank you."

<u>Variation:</u>

- Slice the avocado on the WASA cracker from the previous Liver Treatment. I use a fork and smash it down a little so it doesn't slide off my cracker.

- Add a slice of tomato (optional)

- Sprinkle a little Celtic sea salt and eat

Learning to eat in a simpler way is a good step towards good liver health.

<u>Liver Treatment Eight</u>

Eat cantaloupe or your favorite melon for breakfast

Americans love our cereal and milk. The only problem? Both are dead food. Cereal is in a box and the first two ingredients are normally white, refined sugar and an "ose" word or two that means more sugar. Deadly.

We have already talked about the dangers of cow milk, and thus you have invented the breakfast of fatty liver people. What's that breakfast? We call it cereal.

Eating fresh, raw fruit has a two-fold advantage to extinguish liver disease:

1) builds friendly bacteria that encourages your liver.

2) gives you nutrients your body can easily absorb.

What to do:
- **Rinse the cantaloupe skin.**

- **Cut across the center to make two halves The center of the cantaloupe would be the part that does NOT have the knot. The knot is the top of the cantaloupe.**

- **Scoop out the middle of seeds with a Tablespoon and then throw them out.**

- **Get a spoon and eat out of the bowl that was given to you naturally from the skin.**

- **Breakfast is served faster than any fast food lane in any drive-through restaurant.**

- **Sweet and yummy!**

Loaded with friendly germs and

natural sugar from God to give you energy!

Liver Treatment Nine

Breakfast Smoothie for breakfast

Fruit continues to be the fastest and best combination for breakfast. A breakfast smoothie is tasty and gives you a morning full of friendly germs to jump start your day. YUM – eat those germs. Never take a probiotic (friendly germs) from a pill. It is extremely difficult to receive living germs from a dead pill.

Ingredients:
3 or 4 peeled, ripe bananas
1 cup ice (about 5 cubes)
1 teaspoon EVOO (extra virgin olive oil)

What to do:
Blender:
- **Add peeled banana (half at a time)**
- **Pulse until smooth.**
- **Add EVOO**
- **Add ice.**
- **Pulse until smooth.**
- **Drink cold.**

<u>Liver Treatment Ten</u>

Strawberry Smoothie for Breakfast

Ingredients:
3 or 4 peeled, ripe bananas
1 cup frozen strawberries OR frozen blueberries
1 teaspoon EVOO (extra virgin olive oil)

What to do:
Blender:
- **Add peeled banana (half at a time)**
- **Pulse until smooth.**
- **Add EVOO**

- Add frozen strawberries and pulse until smooth. Strawberry Ingredients should say: Strawberries – that's it.

- Drink cold.

Liver Treatment Eleven

Drink a morning cup of hot water with Unsulphered Blackstrap Molasses

It's simple and it is quick. If you hate it, skip it.

Best Energy Drink:

I drink a hot mug of water with one Tablespoon of Blackstrap Molasses a few mornings a week. It is a great source of a "B" vitamin supplement and is loaded with minerals as well. Please buy the "UN-sulphered" kind.

Liver Treatment Twelve

Add EVOO to your life by using it to sauté veggies

This is a great lunch or dinner:

Ice Box Special:

When my grandmother wanted to clean out the refrigerator, she had a very creative way of fooling us kids that we were getting something to eat that was very special.

We would raid the refrigerator and find all the little bit of this and little bit of that in the refrigerator and sauté it in EVOO for a meal. If she needed more food than she would stuff the leftovers from the fry pan into a flat bread for "Ice Box Wraps!"

What to do:
In an iron skillet:
- Liberally pour in EVOO. About a quarter inch to start. You can always add more later. No, this is NOT greasy. This is food as medicine. EVOO is good for your liver.

- On medium heat, stir all the left over ingredients until they are all warmed through. Have a salad on the side and maybe something from the grill.

- If you need more food, then fry the potatoes first so they can become golden brown and crunchy. They should be raw potatoes and never frozen.

- This takes about 30 minutes with the lid on and the heat at medium to medium high. Never smoke EVOO.

- Add all the ice box special ingredients to the browned potatoes.

- When all ingredients are steaming hot, serve.

Flatbread Variation:

- Warm the flatbread in a different fry pan with some EVOO. I you it crunchy, and fry the bread on both sides.

- Add the cooked ice box special ingredients onto the bread.

- Pour a little EVOO salad dressing on top of everything OR use the EVOO mustard.

- Wrap and eat. Have plenty of napkins close by.

Liver Treatment Thirteen

Eat creamy oatmeal for breakfast

Oatmeal - Creamy

Ingredients into a Blender: Makes two servings:

2 cups of old fashioned oatmeal
1 Tablespoon EVOO
1/3 cup local, raw honey
2.5 cups of filtered water without fluoride

Blend well and equally pour oatmeal mixture immediately into the three servings as this recipe tends to settle in the bottom of the blender fast.

What to do:
In a small, glass or stainless steel pot:
- **Fast Method: (about 4 minutes) Pour one serving into a pot and cook on high heat while constantly stirring the oatmeal. Stir with a Tablespoon and continually scrape the bottom as you stir.**

- When you feel your spoon sticking to the bottom, turn off the heat and stir to the thickness you like OFF THE HEAT.

- Serve with some fruit on the side.

Liver Treatment Fourteen

Popcorn and a movie

At the end of a day, I find it very relaxing to have popcorn and a movie. I like romantic comedies that were produced in the 40's and 50's. Very clean and very relaxing.

I make the popcorn from the recipe in this book. I sometimes make a double recipe of popcorn because it makes a great grab-and-go snack for the next day. I put any leftover popcorn in a gallon freezer bag, I store it on the kitchen counter for a few days. More than two days and the popcorn starts to lose its crunch.

Liver Treatment Fifteen

Drink three glasses of filtered water without fluoride BEFORE lunch.

This is a terrific way to help flush out toxins out of your body. This also helps with easier bowel movements. Small little rocks in the bathroom mean your body is recycling the water from your large intestines because you don't drink enough filtered water without fluoride. Little rocks also mean that your gut may be good bacteria poor. Constipation is more than just eating fiber and drinking water. Constipation is also about a good ecosystem in your small intestines of friendly germs.

All other drinks do NOT count towards this water quota. All other drinks are not as important as drinking water each day. Coffee is not water even though you made it with water. The same for juice – even fresh squeezed.

Filtered water without fluoride is water and nothing else.

Liver Treatment Sixteen

Use EVOO on your skin after you shower,

and

Remove Fluoride from your diet.

Skin softeners are loaded with chemicals. We put them on our face, hands and our entire body. Did you know that your skin can absorb water when you take a bath? A little lavender oil in a hot bath does wonders to relax you because we absorb the lavender and the water from the bath through our skin.

Because of our body's ability to absorb through the skin, I rarely use any store bought skin care products on my skin. I mainly use EVOO. I never use sun screen because of all the chemicals that are put in the creams. I wear a long sleeve shirt and a hat for the Florida sun – a better choice than putting chemicals on your skin or on your child's skin.

I want you to try this treatment after your next shower. No, you won't feel greasy from the EVOO. Your body will absorb the EVOO before it is time for you to put your clothes on.

What to do:
- **Shower.**

- **Towel dry.**

- **Pour a little (about a Tablespoon) of EVOO into the palm of your hand and apply on your body as you would any moisturizing lotion.**

- **That's it. Get dressed as usual.**

- **I do NOT suggest EVOO for aftershave for men. Cold water achieves the same thing – to close the pours.**

Fluoride removal:

- Look at your toothpaste's ingredients. If you have any fake sweeteners listed, please look for another toothpaste.

- Fluoride in your toothpaste should be avoided as well because some research I've read indicates that it will change brain chemistry and destroy your thyroid.

- Fluoride leaches calcium from your bones.

Liver Treatment Seventeen

Turn off your internet router for wifi when you sleep.

Okay, you may think I have gone off my rocker for this Liver Treatment, but this is a real problem for me and disturbs my sleep. Yes, my students have tried this to be beneficial as well. Real Life Story:

I always thought my disturbed sleep was because I type for many hours during the day on my computer. Not willing to give up working on my computer, I tried drinking chamomile tea, and drinking the fermented wine to help my sleep. Did they help? Yes, but I still had dreams of typing on my computer all night long.

Then I got very sick one winter with a horrible flu. My girlfriend went to the doctor three times to get a prescription for antibiotics. This was a very rough bug, and got me so sick I was unable to get out of bed for well over a week.

I started to think, "Why am I still having dreams of working on my computer when I haven't touched my computer for days and days.

I had a hunch, and thought I would try it. I got up and went to the wifi and unplugged it. That night was the first night in many months that I did NOT dream of working on my computer all through the night. Yes, it worked for me.

So, until you try this, please don't think I've lost my mind because this has really helped me sleep better.

Please know:

If you don't have a good night's rest, it is impossible to have good liver health.

Liver Treatment Eighteen

Remove all the electrical wall warts within six feet of where you sleep

This Liver Treatment will improve your sleep. Sleep is a crucial element in your life to obtain better liver health.

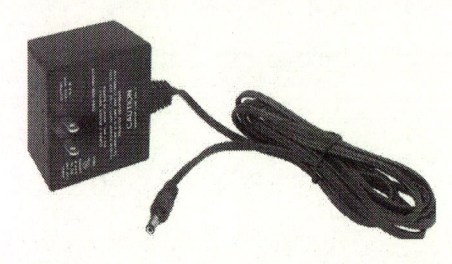

First of all, what are wall warts? No, it is not a disease on your skin. A wall wart is that box that is on the electrical cord on your computer, your clock radio, the stereo, the television, most electrical appliances around the house have one.

Measure all of your wall warts to be at least six feet away from where you lay your head to sleep. This is not a difficult thing to do, but it does take time to check. In fact, putting your clock radio on the table across the room may help you from hitting the snooze button too often.

If your bedroom connects to another room, then go into that room and check the outlets in that room that are on the other side of the room where you lay your head. You can move the wall warts or put them on a power switch that has an on and on button or switch.

The wall warts produce an RF or sound frequency that may interrupt your deep sleep. When you want to use the electrical gadget that is connected to the power strip, you can turn it on easily. I do this with the television that is in my bedroom. Before I go to bed, I turn off the power strip, and it turns off the television. The power strip stays off all the time unless I want to watch the television. This way I do not need to remember to turn it off before I lay down to sleep.

This will help you have a more restful night of sleep and that will translate into better liver health. The article that I read on RF from wall warts said that the electrical waves that come out of the wall wart can prohibit the brain from entering a deeper sleep or "REM" sleep. Without this deep sleep, your body will not be able to give your brain the rest it must have in order to repair your cells and detoxify the liver.

Liver Treatment Nineteen

Eat Almonds on your daily salad.

Almonds are a natural antidepressant. The ingredients on the almonds must say: Almonds. That's it and nothing else.

Dry roasted is best without any oil.

Store almonds in the refrigerator so they won't go rancid. Rancid almonds taste bitter and bad.

Liver Treatment Twenty

Make the grape drink or wine recipe.

Making this recipe will take about twenty minutes of your time and two-to-three days to wait for the natural fermenting to take place. You may want to consider drinking four-to-eight ounces of this friendly bacteria drink every day to help your liver.

This recipe is a giant step towards repopulating the friendly bacteria in your gut.

The Bible has a mention of Paul (he wrote nearly half of the New Testament) writing to his protégé, Timothy to advise him to take a little wine for his upset stomach. The wine that Paul suggested to fix Timothy's indigestion was very similar to the homemade wine recipe that is in this book.

The wine was a remedy because it would add friendly germs to Timothy's tummy and the upset stomach would go away. Hippocrates - who is sometimes considered to be the "Father of Medicine" suggested:

"Let your food be your medicine
Let your medicine be your food."

Liver Treatment Twenty One

Pick one of the soups to make in the crock pot.

This is a fantastic way to make several meals with a small preparation time. Soup is my comfort food. Don't worry about the friendly germs being killed by the crock pot. The opposite is true, the crock pot concentrates the nutrients from the slow cooking, and the fiber in the fresh vegetables holds on to the friendly germ benefits for improved liver function.

This is a perfect time to hire a helper if you are still feeling puny. Any of the soups boost your mood.

Addendum: Adapting your Recipes

Adapting recipes is sometimes difficult because most Americans think they are cooking from scratch when they are really relying on chemicals in their "seasonings" to give their food the flavor they have become accustomed to eating. Like what?

Like mayonnaise in their potato salad. Mayonnaise and most refrigerator-door condiments contain more chemicals than a chemistry set. These chemicals are deadly to the health of your liver. When you don't use store-bought chemicals, the "WOW" taste will be replaced by the taste of real, whole foods. It is still a "WOW" taste, but not at the cost of your liver's health. Some people need a time to transition, most do not.

Please see "Cooking Substitutes" for a mock milk for when you need milk in your recipe. This recipe works well. The mock cream recipe is good, too. Not the taste of cream, but close enough in taste for a recipe The health benefits are great because you will be deleting all of the estrogen and other chemicals fed to a cow here in America that contributes to osteoporosis and other deadly diseases.

The mock white sugar suggestions will help you to adapt recipes that require sugar.

Innocent sounding baking powder has aluminum in it and is not good for a person who wants to know who they are when they become old. Aluminum has been linked by some researchers to Alzheimer's Disease. Alzheimer's disease is a disease of inflammation of the brain. It is my theory that the aluminum contributes to inflammation.

The mock lemon juice ingredient is so simple, you will wonder why you did not think of it yourself.

If you need help adapting one of your recipes, please go to my website and leave me a comment, and I'll see if I can help with any suggestions. http://www.MigrainePhD.com/contact

Addendum: Fruit - the easiest and best breakfast

When you think of the Farmer's Market, this should become your "Farmacy" when your food becomes your medicine.

The "I don't have time for breakfast" club, now has an answer to the dilemma of making time for eating breakfast: Cereal that is "legal" is difficult to find. The only Food Manufacturer to trust is God.

1) Very little time is involved for grabbing a banana as you fly low out the door.

2. No time is involved for eating an apple as you drive to work. The apple is the perfect one-handed meal with a tasty wrapper.

Fruit is:

- Fast.

- Low calorie.

- Portable.

- Fruits are high in water content. The natural water content in fruit is especially formulated by the same Person who formulated you. You have Designer sweet water and Designer food all rolled into one healthy food—fruit!

- Packed with nutrients.

- Fruits are low in fat.

- High in fiber (protects against colon cancer)

- Don't even think about the sugar fruit has might bad for you.

Fruit is truly Food as Medicine because your Creator packaged it!

Benefits of fruit include:

- Helps the body digest fat. (helps you lose weight)
- Helps to cleanse toxins out of the body.
- Fruit satisfies your sweet tooth with God's dessert.

Please NOTE:

Part of losing weight is changing your "wanter". That means you won't "want" junk food anymore because you are into the fruit habit. Fruit will satisfy your sweet tooth, and won't make you fat. Changing a life style is difficult because you are changing the way you think. Once the "thinker" gets changed, the lifestyle follows.

The Bible says,
"As a man thinketh, so he is."

Thoughts are the seeds of actions.
Actions are the seeds of habits.
Habits are the seeds of a lifestyle.

Addendum: Planning a Family Outing

Saturdays are a great day for an outing. It doesn't have to cost money to have fun with your family. With a little planning, you will be surprised how much the fun depends on just being together and less on how much money you spend. Here's an idea how to plan a fun family outing:

On Friday night, the family can eat make plenty of popcorn. I have a glass lid on my iron skillet to watch the popcorn pop. Put the popcorn in a paper bag or baggie for part of Saturday's take-along snack. One per person is good. If you don't have time to pop the popcorn, then bring a piece of fruit. Bananas are a good favorite fruit and economical.

Any of the Muffin recipes are simple to prepare for an on-the-go breakfast. This way, you can get up, grab your muffins, and your lunch and you are out the door quickly.

PBJ sandwiches are a quick lunch to make up on Friday night and put in sandwich bags. Snacks are easy. Use portable snacks that are packaged by God. An example would be an apple and a pear.

Chili is a quick way to use your crock pot for a Saturday dinner. Why? Because the chili is prepared the night before. In the morning take 10 minutes to put the Chili in the crock pot before you dash out the door. This way the Saturday menu was entirely prepared Friday night as a family and might look like this:

The Outing Menu:

- Breakfast: Muffins to go.

- Snack—10:00 a.m: - banana or apple

- Lunch: PBJ and almonds or other nut.

- Snack: 3:00 p.m.—banana or apple

- Dinner: 5:00 p.m.—arrive home after a hard day of playing to a cooked crock pot recipe.

Addendum: Relapse Insurance

Avoiding a relapse is important, but leaky brain syndrome may be a big contributing factor to play in your relapse. Sometimes I'll read a chapter from one of my books and say, "WOW, I forgot I knew that." All humans suffer with "leaky brain syndrome" and review is a wonderful human necessity. Don't feel bad, this is just a fact of our physical make up. Keep doing your best every day, and review often.

Changing eating habits is a difficult process and sometimes the process reverses itself and you get off course without knowing you've done so until you start feeling bad.

Over the years, my students have embraced the liver cleanse way of eating, but soon begin to forget why they started eating this way in the first place – "OH! I was sick?"

One of my student's **liver enzyme test** began to show negative results. She panicked and called me. Here is the list that I gave to her when she needed a little review. You might call this list a **crash course to re-load your brain** when your brain leaks and you forget some important things you used to know.
Read this list over slowly:

Taking any medication – prescription or over-the-counter - is liver toxic. Your liver controls your energy level. A liver that must filter medications, is a body that has less energy!

The more medication you take and the longer time you take it begins to damage the liver. A damaged liver is a dangerous health threat to your liver. If you have less energy, it is your liver's warning sign to you. Take heed when the president of your body sends you this memo.

Forgetting to eat a fresh raw salad every day – no cheese, no meat, no croutons or any foods that is store bought. Keyword here is "RAW." Raw foods give energy. Cooked raw vegetables in your crock pot once a week gives you MORE energy. A farmer's market is the best choice for purchasing raw fruits and vegetables.

Using a store-bought or restaurant made salad dressing should be avoided because pre-made food has additives, coloring and flavor enhancing chemicals in them. All chemicals destroy your liver. Eating EVOO with every meal helps you lose weight.

Eating more than three can goods a week is NOT recommended. Canned goods are packaged in estrogen-laden plastic to protect the food from turning black if it touches the tin can. (my suggestion for a good goal would be to eat zero canned goods per week.)

Eating frozen vegetables more than three servings a week could be damaging your energy. Frozen vegetables are packaged in an estrogen-laden plastic bag to protect the food from freezer burn. (my suggestion for a good goal would be to eat zero frozen vegetables a week)

Suggestion: Try freezing your own vegetables: You wrap the clean, fresh vegetable first with wax paper, and then put it into a freezer bag. This way of freezing vegetables will last for a few months in the freezer. A better choice would be to put the veggie into one of your canning jars and put on the lid. This method takes up a lot more freezer space, but is a better choice than using any plastic.

Eating out without asking what's in the food is a dangerous practice because restaurants are in business to make money from serving you cheap food and marking it up. It is a business. A business that wants to stay in business MUST practice this principle or go out of business.

If you eat meat at a restaurant, chances are high that your meat won't be organic. Restaurants buy special meats that are designed for them. How? My guess is that this food was raised with more hormones to grow faster and with more fat. Fat tastes better than your home meat and now you know why. If you do decide to eat this meat, it should be about the same size as a deck of cards or skip it and eat organic meat at your house.

Eating meat two or three times a day reduces your energy level. Why? Because all meat is difficult to digest. Not just red meat, but ALL meat. Easier digestion will allow your liver to give you increased energy.

Suggestion:

When you eat out, your best bet is to order a RAW salad and bring your home made salad dressing from home. I like bringing a piece of my bread, too. Ahhh, I have the fellowship of my friends or business associates, and I have MY confidence that I won't be sick the next day. YAY!

Eating any food from a box. (no matter if the ingredients "look" healthy may be dangerous to your health because most boxed foods have more than one ingredient. Never eat a boxed food with more than four ingredients.

Eating more than three servings a week of organic dairy – like eggs, yogurt, sour cream may prove to be dangerous to your health. Try the nut cheese or yogurt in this book. A serving is one cup or 8 ounces. All animal products may cause additional labor for a tired liver because of the way the animal was fed. Now your liver must normalize the extra hormones you ate in your meat.

Eating any frozen entrees or dinners is convenient, but not conducive to your health. (This food is packaged in estrogen laden plastic with added chemicals to trick your brain that the food is food.)

Eating too close to bed time may interrupt sleep, and will put on weight. Yes, I said, "WILL." Eating four hours or less should be avoided. If you are starving, eat a small bowl of grapes or other fresh fruit.

Not getting seven hours of sleep will not give your body enough time to repair and rejuvenate itself. Eight hours seems to be average, but I feel better with nine or ten hours of sleep. No, you cannot "catch up" on your sleep on the week end – that's a myth. If you are tired, you need sleep. You know what you need to give up.

If you have wifi (wireless internet) in your home, turn it off at night or put a timer on it so it will shut off and you don't need to remember. Again, your brain is electrical, and this is an electrical device. If this sounds, too crazy to you, just do it and be quiet.

All colorings in drinks is dangerous because according to Dr. Ben F. Feingold, food colorings activate the nervous system. Drinking beverages with food coloring and unknown ingredients can zap your energy and may interrupt your sleep.

Caffeine first thing in the morning is designed to activate the nervous system and give you a kick start. If you cannot survive with enough energy without your caffeine, then your body is yelling, "**HELP**!" You should have energy from the food you eat and not NEED help from caffeine. Drinking more than two or three caffeine drinks in one day is a warning sign your liver is in trouble.

Addendum: Getting a Good Night's Rest

Getting a good night's rest is very important for anyone wanting to be active and happy the next day. As we age, we need more rest. Just because you had energy and only slept six hours a night when you were younger or before you became ill, does NOT mean you can still do the same abuse to your body today. You probably know most of the things on this list, but sometimes reading what you know re-enforces and solidifies doing what you know you should do.

Go to bed to relax and sleep will occur naturally. Try these simple tips.

One hour before bed, take off all the lights in your house except for the one light you will use to read or to sit and relax. This may be a good time to write down goals for tomorrow. (If this stimulates you to start thinking about tomorrow, read a book.) If other family members object, wear sun glasses or quarantine yourself to your bedroom.

Drink one cup of herbal tea like chamomile. (Two cups is NOT better and it may cause you to need a bathroom break in the middle of the night.)

No television, internet or other electronic devices for the last twenty minutes before bedtime. The key word here is "**relax**." I find that reading is relaxing or a quiet conversation. Not a good time for talking about deep subjects or budgeting.

Take a hot bath as preparation for bed. I will add a few drops of lavender oil. Lavender relaxes you. If you take a shower, add a few drops of the lavender oil to a cap full of EVOO and rub on your arms or legs.

Don't wear synthetic fabric pajamas or night gown to bed. Synthetic materials do not breathe. I use cotton sheets and blanket in my bed. Be <u>comfy</u>.

No plastic or PVC furniture in your bedroom. (Plastic outgases estrogen fumes into the air.)

If you wake up to use the bathroom, do NOT turn on any light. A small night light 10-to-20 feet away will light up more than you think. I have a night light in the kitchen, and it lights up my entire house. (I have a small house.) I can easily see my way to the bathroom from the one night light.

About the Author

Contact the author:

http://www.Migrainephd.com/contact/

Scroll down to find the contact form.

Time

My days they run away from me.
More wrinkles on my face to see.
I've asked God for a little gift.
In heaven, I want a face lift.

Diana Jo Rossano lives in Orlando, Florida where she helps her students to feel better by making a few lifestyle changes. Diana enjoys ballroom dancing, ballet, writing and lecturing.

Dr. Rossano made the discovery of eating this way when she suffered with migraine headaches, low thyroid and fibromyalgia. Not wanting a lifetime of taking prescription pain medication, she went back to school to research why she was having pain. The result? Diana became doctor Diana with a Ph.D. in holistic nutrition.

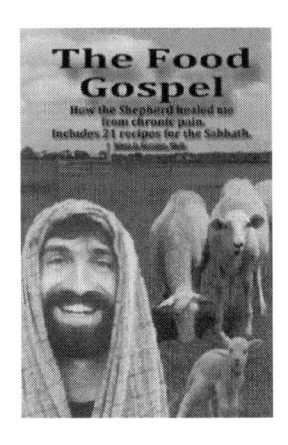

"The Food Gospel" How the Shepherd healed me from chronic pain. Includes 21 recipes for the Sabbath. I honored God with my money, my time, and

I taught Sunday school, but I forgot God at meal time. A great way to understand what the Bible says about food that you may never hear from a pulpit. God wants every part of your life – including the peas on your plate. This book can serve as a group Bible study or used as a quiet time alone with God.

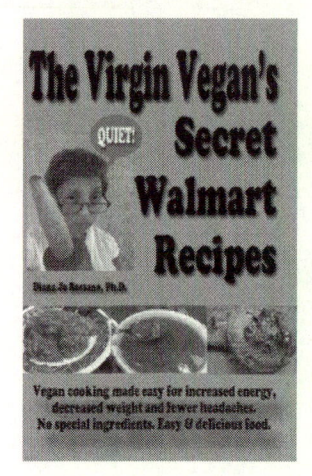

"The Virgin Vegan's Secret Walmart Recipes" Vegan cooking made easy for increased energy, decreased with and fewer headaches. These recipes are liver friendly. No special ingredients. Easy & delicious food. More liver friendly recipes.

This is the perfect place to find all of Dr. Rossano's recipes from her other books that have been made vegan. Why vegan? Because Diana did some research about hormones in her meat and came up that vegan was the next logical step for her to take towards improved health.

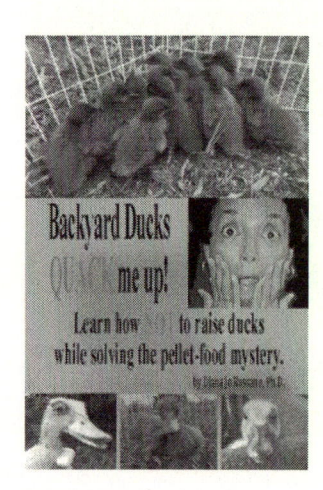

Read Dr. Diana's Duck completed Research in this book or read the complete research below.

"Backyard Ducks QUACK me up! Learn how to NOT raise ducks while solving the pellet-food mystery." This book is not only for raising ducks, but it is also Dr. Diana's research that pointed to her becoming a vegan. Dr. Rossano bought 20 ducklings to raise her own backyard eggs without eating pellet food. To her surprise a mystery arose and her ducks began to die. The research revealed why the ducks died, and that reason convinced her vegan was the way to live. Not like vegans in the U.S., but a virgin vegan without additives and preservatives.

Bibliography

Abrahamson, E. M., M.D., Body, Mind and Sugar, (Holt, Rinehart and Winston, Inc., New York) 1977

Allison, Linda, Blood and Guts, A Working Guide to Your Own Insides, (Little, Brown and Company, Covelo) 1976

Batmangelidj, F., M.D., "Your Body's Many Cries For Water." Global Health Solutions, Inc., Falls Church, Va. 22043, USA. Telephone: 703-848-2333 1992

Barrett, Stephen, M.D. and Jarvis, William T., Ph.D., The Health Robbers, A Close Look at Quackery in America, (Prometheus Books, New York) 1993

Blaylock, Russell L., M.D., Excitotoxins: the Taste that Kills, (Health Press, Santa Fe) 1997

Center for Science in the Public Interest, Safe Food, Eating Wisely in a Risky World, (Living Planet Press, Los Angeles) 1991

Cheraskin, Emmanuel, M.D., D.M.D., Psycho-dietetics, Food as the Key to Emotional Health, (Stein and Day /Publishers/Scarborough House, Briarcliff Manor) 1974

Coca, Arthur F., M.D. "The Pulse Test" (St. Martin's Press, New York) 1956

Contreras, Francisco, M.D., Health in the 21st Century, Will Doctors Survive? (Interpacific Press, Chula Vista) 1997

Feingold, Ben F. M.D., Why Your Child Is Hyper-active, (Random House, New York) 1974

Gaynor, Mitchell L, M.D., Dr. Gaynor's Cancer Prevention Program, (Kensington Books, New York) 1999

Gerson, Max, M.D., A Cancer Therapy, (Gerson Institute, New York) 1958

Green, Joey, Paint Your House with Powdered Milk, (Hiperion, New York) 1996

Haas, Elson M., M.D., Staying Healthy with Nutrition, (Celestial Arts, Berkeley) 1992

Harrington, Geri, Fake Food, Real Food, and Everything in between, Macmillan Publishing Company, Inc., New York) 1987

Heinerman, John, Heinerman's Encyclopedia of Fruits, Vegetables and Herbs (Parker Publishing Company, West Nyack) 1988

Lee, John R., What Your Doctor May Not Tell You About Menopause, (Warner Books, Inc., New York) 1996

Low, Rodolfo, "Migraine, the Breakthrough Study" (Henry Holt & Company, Inc., New York) 1987

MacDonald Baker, Sidney, M.D., Detoxification & Healing, The Key to Optimal Health, (Keats Publishing, Inc., New Canaan) 1997

Manahan, William, M.D., Eat for Health. (H.J. Kramer, Inc., Tiburon) 1988

Mendelsohn, Robert S., M.D., How to Raise a Healthy Child... In spite of your Doctor, (Contemporary Books, Inc., Chicago) 1984

Milunsky, Aubrey, M.D., Choices Not Chances, (Little, Brown, Boston) 1989

National Health Federation Newsletter, Post Office Box 688, Monrovia, California 91017, Phone: 626-357-2181

Pfeiffer, Carl C., Mental and Elemental Nutrients, (Keats Publishing, Inc. New Canaan) 1975

Pinckney, Cathey, & Edward R., M.D., Do-it-yourself Medical Testing, (Facts On File, Inc, New York) 1989

Price, Weston, D.D.S., Nutrition and Physical Degeneration, (Keats Publishing, Inc., New Canaan) 1939, 1-800-366-3748

Pritikin, Nathan, Diet for Runners, (A Fireside Book, New York) 1985

Randolph, Theron G., M.D., An Alternative Approach to Allergies, (Harper & Row, New York) 1979

Reuben, David, M.D., Everything You Always Wanted to Know About Nutrition, (Simon and Schuster, New York) 1978

Ross, Harvey M., M.D. & Saunders, Jeraldine, Hypoglycemia: The Disease Your Doctor Won't Treat (Pinnacle Books, New York) 1990

Rowan, Robert L., M.D., How to Control High Blood Pressure without Drugs, (Charles Scribner's Sons, New York) 1986

Schwartz, George R. M.D. "In Bad Taste, The MSG Syndrome," A Signet Book, New American Library, A division of Penguin Books, USA, Inc. 1988

Steinman, David, Living Healthy in a Toxic World, (A Perigee Book, New York) 1996

Theodosakis, Jason, M.D., The Arthritis Cure, (St Martin's Griffin, New York) 1997

Turner, Dorothy, Milk, (Wayland (Publishers) Ltd., Hove, East Sussex) 1988

Vigilante, Kevin, M.D., Low-Fat Lies, High-Fat Frauds, (LifeLine Press, Washington, DC) 1999

Weeks, Nora, The Medical Discoveries of Edward Bach Physician, (The C. W. Daniel Company Limited, Essex) 1973

Weil, Andrew, M.D. Health and Healing, (Houghton Mifflin Company, Boston, New York) 1983

Winters, Ruth, A Consumer's Dictionary of Food Additives, (Three Rivers Press, New York) 1994

Wright, Jonathan V, M.D., Nutrition and Healing, (Newsletter) Agora South, L.L.C., 819 N. Charles St. Baltimore, MD. 21201, Phone: 978-514-7851

Wootan, George, M.D., "Take Charge of Your Child's Health," (Marlowe and Co., New York) 2000

Index for Recipes

Almond Milk 202
Ants 373
Apple Butter 203
Avoiding a relapse 411
Baby Powder or Foot Powder: 373
Baked Beans 294
Baked Potato 295
Banana Bread 229
Banana Bread Secret 231
Basic Dietary Goals 26
Batter Mix for Frying 205
Bean Dip 205
Beans and Rice Casserole 249
Beef 262
Beef-broth Vegetable Soup 245
Best Energy Drink: 393
Biscuits 260
Blackstrap Molasses 359, 393
Bran Muffins 241
Bread 255, 296, 312, 315, 317, 322
Bread Crumbs 207
Bread Rolls 260
Bread Sticks 258
Bread variations 258
Brown Rice 308
Brownie Recipe (Mock) 229
Brownies (Mock) 229
Bruschetta Gargoyle Bread 296
Bug Bites 373
buyer beware!! 301
caffeine quiz 112
Candied Carrots 297
Candied Yams 298
Carrot Bread 234
Carrot Cake 232
Carrot Muffins 233
Carrot Sheet Cake 234
CAUTION for Milk Thistle 25
Chicken 275

Chicken and Yellow Rice	248
Chicken Broth	208
Chicken Broth Gravy	209
Chicken Pasta Creole	246
Chicken Salad Sandwiches	300
Chicken Soup (Creamy)	299
Chicken Soup Base	209
Chili	243
Chinese Mustard	367
Chocolate Cake	324
Chocolate Frosting	232
Cholesterol Test	94
chronic stone former	359
Cinnamon Buns	258
Cocoa (Hot)	367
Condiments and Chemicals	123
Constipation	397
Cook Ahead Meatloaf and 3 more meals	341
Cook Ahead Meatloaf II for Freezing	343
Cook Ahead Mock Sausage Meat	340
Cook Ahead Shredded Chicken	344
Cookies - Graham	327
Cookies - Nut Raisin	330
Cookies - Oatmeal Raisin	329
Cookies - Protein	336
Cookies Peanut Butter	334
Corn and Potato Casserole	302
Corn Bread	311
Corn Bread Stuffing	303
Corn silk tea	358
Cornstarch	373
crash course to re-load your brain	411
cut garlic	219
Deodorant	373
Depression & other emotional symptoms:	359
Dessert - Spinach Pie	337
Dessert - Stuffed Dates	338
Dessert - Sweet Potato Pie	339
Dinner Rolls	260
Dr. B's Recipe	345
Dr. Castelli - Heart Disease	139

Drain Cleaner...374
Drain Freshener 374
Dressing 213, 214
Drink Choices..357
Drink Dandelion Tea 361
dumb 360
Ease the Pressure Tips 112
eating at a salad bar 385
eating out technique..192
Egg Salad 305
EVOO Mayonnaise..220
EVOO Mustard 221
EVOO Salad Dressing 214
Family Outing...409
Filtered water without fluoride: 362
first loaf of Organic Bread 317
Fish and Chips 250
Flatbread 312
Fluoride...398
French Dressing 213
French Toast 234
friendly germs are responsible for 143
Frittata...228
Fruit Dessert Layered 328
Fryer 201
Gargle 374
Garlic EVOO 367
Garlic Oil..213, 367
Grandma's Molasses 360
Granola..235
Grape Soda or Grape Wine 363
Grapes Warning...365
Gravy...209
Grilled Cheese 251
Guacamole...215
Hair Dye Warning 374
Hair Frizzes 375
Herbal Liver Medicine 377
Hollandaise Sauce 216
Home Canning Information..346
Home made syrup:..266

Homemade Deep Fryer	201
homemade parsley	130
how I knead bread	256
How much dressing should you use?	385
How to cut garlic	219
How to Dry Parsley	129
How to pick an avocado:	389
Hummus	217
I are dumb:	360
Ice Box Special:	393
improve your sleep	400
Index for Recipes	427
Irish Soda Bread	322
Jambalaya	252
Jelly	219
laboratory rats	104, 172
Lamb Stew	253
Lazy Bread	255
Lazy Bread variations	258
Lazy Sunday	272
Lemon Peel Tea	368
Lemonade Mix	368
liver enzyme test	411
Liver Treatment Eight	390
Liver Treatment Eighteen	400
Liver Treatment Eleven	393
Liver Treatment Fifteen	396
Liver Treatment Five	386
Liver Treatment Four	384
Liver Treatment Fourteen	396
Liver Treatment Nine	391
Liver Treatment Nineteen	401
Liver Treatment One	381
Liver Treatment Seven	388
Liver Treatment Seventeen	398
Liver Treatment Six	387
Liver Treatment Sixteen	397
Liver Treatment Ten	392
Liver Treatment Thirteen	395
Liver Treatment Three	382
Liver Treatment Twelve	393

Liver Treatment Twenty 402
Liver Treatment Twenty One 402
Liver Treatment Two 382
Love Your Liver 381
Macaroni Salad 306
Mashed Potatoes 306
Mayonnaise 220
Meat Recommendations 371
Meatloaf 262
Mexican Pan Bread 236
Mexican Stir Fry 264
Milk 202
Milk Thistle 377
Minced Garlic 218
Mock Baking Powder 369
Mock Breakfast Sausage 238
Mock Cream (for cooking 369
Mock Italian Sausage 239
Mock Jelly 219
Mock Lemon Juice 370
Mock Milk (for cooking 369
Mock Mustard 221
Mock Play Dough 375
Mock White Sugar (in recipes 370
Monosodium Glutamate Aliases: 125
Mushrooms 309
Mustard 221
Nut Yogurt 353
Oatmeal - Creamy 395
Okra and Tomatoes 307
Organic Bread 315
Organic Bread Step Three or 317
Organic Bread Step Two 316
Organic Bread, Second Loaf 319
Outing Menu: 409
Pancakes 265
Paper Mache 375
Party 379
Pasta Primavera 266
Peanut Butter 240
Peppers and Yellow Rice 269

Peppers and Yellow Rice Casserole 268
Perfect Brown Rice 308
Pickles 221
Pie Crust - Nutty 331
Pie Crust - Rolled Oats 333
Pie Crust Two 332
Pizza Crust (Thin) 321
Pizza Delivery 40
Pizza Dough 261
Pizza Topping 271
Popcorn 350
Popcorn Popper Review 351
Pre-heating oven 39
Pretzel Dough 261
Promoting Digestion 357
Protein Myth 371
Real Life Story 31, 37, 50, 59, 64, 76, 144, 226, 399
Recipe Section 199
Red Beans and Rice 272
Red Sauce 212
Salad bar no – no's 385
Salad Dressing 214
Salmon Italian Style 273
Salmon Patties 274
Salsa (Cooked) 223
Salsa (Raw) 222
Salt Example 69
Santa Fe Chicken 275
Sauce in ten minutes 211
Sausage 238
secret 231
Sheet-Cake 326
Simple Salad Dressing 384
Sloppy Joes 276
Smoothie 242
Snack - Bean Sprouts 348
Snack - Popcorn 350
Snack - Popcorn Treat 352
Spaghetti Sauce (Crock) 277
Spaghetti Sauce (Oven) 279
Stainless Steel Cleaner: 375

Stir Fry 281
Store-bought bread? 301
Strained Tomatoes 224
Strained Tomatoes Okay Food Option #2 225
Stress 73
Stuffed Mushrooms 309
Stuffed Peppers 282
Stuffing 303
Substitutes More 373
Sweet Potato Pie 339
Tabouleh 310
Texas Fries 283
Tile Cleaner: 376
Tomato Potato Soup 284
Tomato Soup (Creamy) 286
Turkey 287
Vegetable Soup 291
Vegetable Soup Base 227
Veggie Casserole 289
WASA Ingredients: 387
Water Requirement 39
Window & Counter Top Cleaner: 376
Wine or Grape Juice Basics 362
yeast free bread 255
yeast-free bread 315
Yoghurt 353
Yogurt 353
Yummy Pockets I 292
Yummy Pockets II 293
Yummy Pockets III 294

Made in the USA
Middletown, DE
26 January 2017